1996

ETHICAL CHOICES

ETHICAL CHOICES
Case Studies
for Medical Practice

Lois Snyder, JD, Editor
American College of Physicians
Philadelphia, Pennsylvania

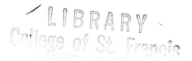
AMERICAN COLLEGE OF PHYSICIANS
PHILADELPHIA, PENNSYLVANIA

A|C|P

Acquisitions Editor: Mary K. Ruff
Director of Book and Journal Publishing: Pamela Fried
Production Supervisor: Patricia C. Walter
Interior Design: Patricia C. Walter
Cover Design: Colleen Woods-Esposito

Printed in the United States of America.

Composition by *Christine H. Poullain.*
Printing/binding by *Capital City Press.*
Cover printed by *Capital City Press.*

American College of Physicians
Independence Mall West
Sixth Street at Race
Philadelphia, PA 19106-1572

> *A version of each case history presented herein has been published previously in the* ACP Observer, *from 1990 to January 1996.*

Library of Congress Cataloging in Publication Data

Ethical choices : case studies for medical practice / Lois Snyder.
    129 p.   cm.
    Includes bibliographical references and index.
    ISBN 0-943126-43-6
    1. Medical ethics—Case studies.   I. Snyder, Lois, 1961-
R724.E784 1996
174′.2—dc20
                                                    96-5405
                                                    CIP

96 97 98 99 00 01 / 9 8 7 6 5 4 3 2 1

To my daughter Hannah,
who makes it all clear.

CONTRIBUTORS

Anne-Marie Audet, MD
Medical Research Associate
American College of Physicians
Philadelphia, Pennsylvania
(from September 1991 to January 1994)

Troyen A. Brennan, MD, JD, MPH, FACP
Professor of Medicine
Harvard Medical School
Professor of Law and Public Health
Harvard School of Public Health
Boston, Massachusetts

Errol D. Crook, MD
Assistant Professor of Medicine
Division of Nephrology
University of Mississippi Medical Center
Jackson, Mississippi

Frank Davidoff, MD, FACP
Senior Vice President, Education
American College of Physicians
Philadelphia, Pennsylvania
(from July 1987 to March 1995)
Editor, *Annals of Internal Medicine*
American College of Physicians
Philadelphia, Pennsylvania

Kathleen L. Egan, PhD
Senior Associate for Research and Development
American College of Physicians
Philadelphia, Pennsylvania

Alan L. Hillman, MD, MBA, FACP
Director, Center for Health Policy
Leonard Davis Institute of Health Economics
Associate Professor of Medicine and
    Health Care Management
School of Medicine and The Wharton School
University of Pennsylvania
Philadelphia, Pennsylvania

Lois Snyder, JD
Ethics and Health Policy Counsel
American College of Physicians
Philadelphia, Pennsylvania

Susan W. Tolle, MD, FACP
Director, Center for Ethics in Health Care
Oregon Health Sciences University
Portland, Oregon

Janet Weiner, MPH
Research Associate
American College of Physicians
Philadelphia, Pennsylvania
(from July 1989 to March 1995)

CONTENTS

PREFACE

The case studies in this collection were developed from 1990 to 1995 under the auspices of the American College of Physicians Ethics Committee, which in 1994 became the Ethics and Human Rights Committee. The commentaries expand on principles contained in College policy, mostly as found in the College's *Ethics Manual*. Work has already begun on a fourth edition of the manual.

Topic selection was either staff-, committee-, or ACP member–driven and was based on common ethical problems in medical practice. This book is by no means comprehensive. Because the case study series is ongoing, comments and topic ideas from the reader are encouraged.

An annotated bibliography was added to each case study in mid-1995. The purpose of the bibliography is to bring each case up-to-date and to guide the reader to the latest and best sources of information on each topic. All articles cited can be found in readily available medical journals.

I originally conceived the case study series with three goals in mind: first, to make principles more relevant to daily medical practice by discussing their application in specific situations; second, to make the reader think about issues that are important but, being largely the stuff of everyday medical encounters, often are not glamorous and as such are ones that might not otherwise command much explicit attention; and third, to demonstrate medical ethics in action while considering the real motivations behind behavior. I hope that these purposes have been achieved on some level for practitioners, patients, students, and policymakers. I also hope that the book is a good read.

Lois Snyder, JD
American College of Physicians

FOREWORD

In recent years, debate has begun in the field of medical ethics concerning frameworks for the discussion and analysis of problems in medical ethics. Rather than starting exclusively from assumptions about ethics drawn from historical values of the profession, such as the Hippocratic oath, or universal rules, such as "always prolong life" or "never tell a lie," philosophers have articulated ways in which different values paradigms may result in different approaches to resolving specific ethical dilemmas. For example, traditional frameworks included various "rule-based ethics," whereas nontraditional ones claimed that "situation ethics" was more relevant to real-life situations. Situation ethics allows the specific circumstances to influence the rule; for example, a patient suffering from severe depression is not given the complete information about a new diagnosis of cancer until the depression has been successfully treated. New debates have added feminist ethics, historical or social contexts for ethics, and others as well.

This book recognizes that, for physicians, a case-based approach to problem solving is a traditional and time-proven way of addressing problems in medicine. Those of us who have taught ethics on the wards at the bedside, in the outpatient setting, and in the nursing home know that using individual cases in all their complexity is the most effective way to teach medical ethics to medical students and residents. We believe that the case-based approach is the key to understanding medical ethics but that the clinical case for ethics requires a fuller "story" for the values at stake to be understood.

Kathryn Hunter describes the physician's way of thinking in her book *Doctors' Stories*, which was published in 1994. In it she recounts the experience of witnessing numerous medical rounds during which cases were presented by trainees. A Socratic form of analysis was used by attending physicians to help elicit an approach to discovering the patient's diagnosis and determining the best approach to management. Hunter compares this process in medicine to that of Sherlock Holmes in his legendary pursuit of the solutions to mysteries: Holmes would piece together disparate information to create a story, and the story, when it became lucid and credible, became a compelling explanation for a series of otherwise mysterious occurrences. Thus, it is the "stories" that tell us most about the complexity of the interaction of medical practice and conflicts or moral dilemmas. In this book, the case study as "story" is used to best advantage.

Stories are the basis for learning about practical ethical problems in medicine. They provide the foundation on which abstract analysis can and should be grounded. The commentaries that accompany the cases in this book permit the reader to better understand both the substantive issues raised by specific cases and how to formulate a sustained rationale for an ethical argument. In the real world of medical practice, it is the outcome of the story that matters. In the real world of medical ethics, what matters is the assessment of a particular action, or the evaluation of someone's conduct, as well as the rationale that can be supplied in support of the moral assessment or evaluation.

A key reason that ethical issues in health care are so riveting and compelling is they illustrate how real people in real-world situations make hard choices about important matters. *Ethical Choices* takes full advantage of the richness of the clinical setting.

One especially troubling flaw in many writings on medical ethics is that they tend to focus almost exclusively on dilemmas raised by the practice of highly specialized forms of medicine that are often at the frontiers of innovation and technology. For every article written about the ethics of telling a patient the truth about the diagnosis, there are at least as many, and maybe more, about the ethics of using baboon hearts as bridges to transplants that use human hearts obtained from cadaver donors. This book provides a broader perspective to the narrow focus of much of bioethical writing by taking clinical practice and experience seriously. The office, the nursing

home, the ambulatory care clinic, and the Urgi-clinic are as likely to
be locales in which ethical issues arise as are the intensive care unit
or the transplant suite. Furthermore, patients need not be on the
verge of death or critical illness to confound the doctor with difficult
ethical puzzles.

This book also points the reader toward the need to understand
how good ethics and good medical practice go hand in hand. All
too often, ethics is seen as somehow at odds with or an obstacle to
what the doctor's training and judgment require. It is true that ethical concerns are raised only when courses of conduct are suggested that deviate somewhat from what is widely practiced or when a
breach in standard practice is proposed. However, it is not at all
true that ethics is only of interest when something outside the main-
stream of medical practice is contemplated. As many of the cases in
this book make very clear, the clinical practice of medicine is never
very far removed from its normative moral base. Doing good and
avoiding harm are such essential components of medicine that
skillful medical practice requires a physician who is thoughtful and
reflective about how to apply knowledge and skills to particular
instances of disease, illness, anxiety, or disability, be they ordinary
or extraordinary.

Experienced physicians in practice will find this book useful
because it moves from real experience to theoretical analysis, rather
than beginning with theory. Students will find it useful because it is
how they learn in medicine. The book spans the spectrum from dra-
matic life-and-death decision making to moral problems that arise
in the interactions of everyday practice, such as economic conflicts
and relationships with peers. None of these problems are simple,
nor can they be adequately examined by appeal to rules.
Nonetheless, guidelines and principles of medical practice as articulated by the American College of Physicians in its widely cited
Ethics Manual are the basis for the resolution of these cases.
Together, the two resources provide a firm basis for medical ethics
in modern practice.

Ethical Choices belongs on every practitioner's bookshelf. It is a
compelling cornucopia of clinical conundrums and everyday
dilemmas thoughtfully presented and carefully scrutinized. Those

who worry that too much of bioethics is done from the perspective of the armchair will find no reason for concern in these pages. The case material is timely and detailed, and the commentaries and advice are practical and down to earth. Health care professionals looking for useful advice about the daily moral life of medical practice will find good insight in the case studies written by Lois Snyder and colleagues.

Christine K. Cassel, MD
Chair of the Henry L. Schwartz
Deparment of Geriatrics and
Adult Development, Mt Sinai
Medical Center

Arthur L. Caplan, PhD
Director of the University of
Pennsylvania Center for
Bioethics

ACKNOWLEDGMENTS

Thanks are owed to the contributors to this collection of case studies and to the individuals who have served and who currently serve on the American College of Physicians Ethics and Human Rights Committee, who have helped guide the development of the series. Past Committee chairs are Edwin P. Maynard, MD, MACP, and Christine K. Cassel, MD, FACP. Lloyd W. Kitchens Jr., MD, FACP, is the current chair. Past committee members are Elias Abrutyn, MD, FACP; Troyen A. Brennan, MD, JD, MPH, FACP; Richard J. Carroll, MD; Cynthia L. Clagett, MD; Karen E. Coblens, MD; Errol D. Crook, MD; Lee J. Dunn, Jr., Esq.; Carola Eisenberg, MD; Arthur W. Feinberg, MD, FACP; Bernard Lo, MD, FACP; Steven Miles, MD; John A. Mitas II, MD, FACP; Gail Povar, MD; William A. Reynolds, MD, FACP; Gerald E. Thomson, MD, FACP; and Susan W. Tolle, MD, FACP.

Christine K. Cassel, MD, FACP, and Arthur L. Caplan, PhD, are due special thanks for their review of the manuscript and helpful comments, reflections, and guidance. Gratitude is also expressed to Paula S. Katz, Executive Editor, and her staff at *ACP Observer*, in which the case studies were originally published; to Pamela Fried and her staff in the Publishing Division of the American College of Physicians, especially Patricia C. Walter, Production Supervisor; and to Patricia Wieland, expert copy editor. I am also indebted to Linda J. Harris for word processing many iterations of the case studies, to Sharon Hart for bibliographic article retrieval, and to Sharon and Tom Shotkin for assistance in preparing the manuscript.

And, for always, my love and thanks to Hannah, my daughter. At age two years, she is not (yet) a critical reviewer, but she is a source of inspiration, perspective, and joy and of insights I had once forgotten or never fully knew.

Lois Snyder, JD

1

Introduction to Medical Ethics

LOIS SNYDER, JD

Medical ethics has come of age. No longer is it the exclusive province of philosophers, theologians, theoreticians, or medical and legal academicians. Many medical ethics issues—from AIDS dilemmas to doctor–patient sexual relationships, physician-assisted suicide to the withholding or withdrawal of life support—are very much on the minds of practitioners, patients, policymakers, and the media.

Medical ethicists have joined the ranks of talk show guests and news article commentators. This celebrity is good. Talk is good. But in the realm of ethics, talk is mostly important to the extent that it leads to action—the appropriate action.

This collection of case studies is directed toward action: What did the physician do right or wrong; what should she or he do in a given situation? Principles are pondered, abstractions are analyzed, theory is thought through, arguments are articulated—good arguments are critical to practicing good medical ethics. But in the end, in addition to showing *how* to make ethical decisions in the practice of medicine, guidance about *what* constitutes the best ethical course in particular circumstances is provided in most instances.

The issues contemplated in these case studies are pertinent to the health, welfare, and rights of patients as well as to the everyday practice of physicians and physicians-to-be. Patients and their physicians—and the relationships they develop or hope to develop—are under increasing pressure because of changes in health care financing and delivery, technological advancement, the law, and demographic shifts. Although gene therapy, animal-to-human organ transplantation, and other highly controversial issues often shine in the bioethics limelight, more routine issues like the financial incentives inherent in fee-for-service medicine versus managed care, the impaired doctor, and patient preferences for referrals are often more relevant for practitioners and their patients. These case studies examine frequent bedside clinical issues and common issues in professional medical ethics.

What is medical ethics? First, what is ethics? Webster's dictionary defines the term as a theory or system of moral values. I define ethics as what we should do and why. It is also about the sorts of traits and qualities people ought to have or ought to strive to have—the old-fashioned but never out of fashion notion of virtue, of good being done by good people. It is not merely about what you feel in your gut is right or wrong, although this is often a good starting point. It is not just philosophical principles and ideals and rigorous arguments, although these are a large part of doing ethics. It is not only about what the law, a set of socially determined moral minimums, or tradition require. It is about all of these things. But it is never simply a matter of consensus. You cannot just vote to determine what is ethical, although if families, schools, the law, politics, the professions, religion, and culture are doing their jobs, you may happen upon an ethically valid vote.

Bioethics encompasses ethical dilemmas in health care, medicine, and the life sciences, combining both theory and practice. Bioethics as a field is still relatively young, with its formal beginnings in the 1960s and 1970s. Responses to research scandals of the day, such as the Tuskegee syphilis "study," plus a series of reports issued by the President's Commission for the Study of Ethical Problems in Medicine and Biomedical and Behavioral Research on diverse topics such as informed consent, access to health care, genetic screening, and the refusal of life-sustaining treatment helped to lay a foundation for the field. Those issues are still very much alive, along with others raised by scientific advances, changing modes of health care delivery, more knowledgeable and demanding patient-consumers, and developments in law, politics, economics, and culture.

For most patients most of the time, bioethics means medical ethics—the care that they receive from their doctors, the science and art of science that directly touches their lives. If ethics is the soul of medicine then the physician–patient relationship is surely the soul of medical ethics.

Two key principles guide all medical ethics inquiries, especially those involving interactions between physician and patient: beneficence, the duty to do good and act in the best interest of others, and non-maleficence, the duty to do no harm. More recently, two additional principles have been added by many to the bioethical equation: respect for autonomy—the individual's right of bodily self-determination—and justice, with a focus on consideration of fair treatment and distribution of resources.

A listing of principles alone, however, will not take you very far down the road of thoughtful ethical inquiry. For example, many commentators invoke patient autonomy as the key, or sometimes only, aspect of their argument supporting euthanasia or physician-assisted suicide. But they fail to consider the ethical, moral, and social heart of the matter they raise: Autonomy for what? What are the purposes and consequences of such self-determination? Euthanasia and physician-assisted suicide are complex issues. There are good arguments to make in response to the above questions and to other aspects of these issues. Arguments that rely on mantras, however, are not helpful.

After all is said, something must be done. Individuals must be aware of ethical issues in health care, confront them, reason through them, and then act. Good bioethics provides good reasons for action. For example, when a physician makes a mistake and does not follow up on a test result, there are principles at stake, and more important to the patient, there are consequences. The physician must act as an ethical and moral matter, and she or he must act as a practical matter, lest she or he be acted upon (by, for example, a malpractice attorney or a disciplinary body). When a potential new Medicaid patient or patient with HIV shows up at the doctor's door, the doctor must decide whether to accept the person as a patient. When a patient wants care that the physician thinks is not medically necessary or appropriate, the doctor must decide what to do and say and the patient must decide how to respond.

Much of what many physicians already do without detailed reflection in many clinical encounters is based on what I think is an intuitive sense about what is ethical and appropriate in a given situation, part of a mindset and worldview born of the culture of medicine and, perhaps, the character and values of the men and women who choose medicine as their profession and life. With millions of clinical encounters occurring each day, ethical problems are not derailing patient care.

With that said, there is still plenty of room for refinement and improvement. The culture of medicine has also had its downside. A notable example is the profession's collective behavior in the bad old days before the firm establishment in physician consciousness of the concepts of full disclosure, informed consent, and shared patient–physician decision making—where appropriate. For some patients, a decision about decision making means requesting not to be told all the details and granting authority to the doctor to climb the decision tree alone. And there are, of course, appropriate limits to the care a patient may demand, although defining those limits is thought by some to be among the hardest tasks in bioethics today.

Physician practice instincts infuse medical ethics deliberations with judgment, passion, compassion, hope, bias, and more—the elements, after all, that cause people to act. We need to consider these very real aspects of what people do and why in considerations of ethics problems. Analysis of these motives and resultant actions provides another reason for the case study format here. Just as most law arises in the context of specific cases with specific fact patterns, cases can provide a foundation for practical medical ethics. In addition, a dry analysis of principles devoid of meaningful context probably does not motivate a busy practitioner or intellectually stressed student to finish reading the page on which it is written, let alone incorporate ethics into the way he or she acts or feels. Case studies as an ethics education tool, especially cases about common problems, can potentially help make more behavior more right, more deliberate, and to the proper extent, more rational.

But not too rational. Principles and rules, whether about substance or procedure, are not moral actors. We are.

PART I

The Patient and Physician: The Clinical Encounter

The patient–physician relationship—it is how patients seek care and comfort and a large element of why many physicians practice medicine. The relationship entails rights and responsibilities, both ethical and legal, for the physician and patient—an obvious but central guiding fact. Care is a joint endeavor.

Many types of clinical encounters could serve as the basis for thought-provoking case studies. Part I highlights aspects of two care issues for two important groups of patients: the dying and the elderly. Chapters 2 and 3 discuss the timely issue of physician-assisted suicide, including arguments for and against and their implications in Chapter 2 and more direct care issues in Chapter 3. Chapter 4 examines the growing concern over elder neglect.

2

Physician-Assisted Suicide

Commentary by LOIS SNYDER, JD
Case History by JANET WEINER, MPH

CASE HISTORY

Ella Washington, age 60, visits Dr. Jones, her internist for the past 20 years. She describes her symptoms— nausea, stomach pain, and weight loss—to the doctor. The workup shows the presence of pancreatic cancer that has metastasized to the liver.

Dr. Jones and Ms. Washington talk extensively about her diagnosis, poor prognosis, and the lack of curative therapies. In response to her direct question, Dr. Jones tells Ms. Washington that she probably has less than six months to live. He refers her to an oncologist for further examination and advice and schedules her for another appointment to review the situation.

Continued

7

Ms. Washington returns in a few weeks, accompanied by her husband and son. She has consulted the oncologist and seems to have a clear understanding of her condition. Her family appears supportive as they talk about palliative therapies and home hospice care.

Before Ms. Washington leaves, she tells Dr. Jones that she wants to "die with dignity" and needs to be able to take her own life in the least painful way possible when the time comes. She says that she has spoken to her family at length and that they support her decision. She claims that fear of a painful, lingering death will prevent her from enjoying her remaining time. She tells Dr. Jones that she obtained information from the Hemlock Society on methods of suicide and bought a copy of *Final Exit* by the society's executive director. She asks Dr. Jones to prescribe barbiturates.

Dr. Jones refuses Ms. Washington's request but asks her to return to see him in a few weeks after she consults with a psychiatrist to verify that she is not significantly depressed. She complies and returns to Dr. Jones' office a few weeks later with the same prescription request. "This is my decision," she says firmly. "We've known each other a long time. I trust you; but if you don't help me, I'll find someone who will, or I'll do it myself. Please don't make this harder on me and my family."

She explains that the security of having enough barbiturates to commit suicide, when and if the time comes, would allow her to live fully and enjoy the present. Dr. Jones is convinced that Ms. Washington is not despondent and is thinking rationally. They agree to meet regularly, and she promises to consult with him before taking her life. Dr. Jones then writes the prescription for barbiturates.

The next four months are fulfilling for Ms. Washington, although she tires easily and has some pain. She spends time with her husband and son and renews and reinforces old friendships. She endures intermittent physical and emotional hardships but seems to bounce back from periods of sadness and anger.

Then she becomes weaker, and the nausea and stomach pain grow more constant and acute. Despite extensive efforts to minimize her discomfort, she feels that the immediate future holds what she fears most: increased pain, dependence, and disability. As agreed, she meets with Dr. Jones to inform him that she will soon commit suicide. Two days later, Ms. Washington's husband calls Dr. Jones to say that she died at home after saying good-bye to her family and closest friends.

———⟫•◆•⟪———

COMMENTARY

Background

After Jack Kevorkian, MD, enabled Janet Adkins to end her life in 1990 using the "suicide machine" he had set up in his Volkswagen van, attention centered on the fact that Dr. Kevorkian did not have a long-standing patient–physician relationship with Ms. Adkins, who had Alzheimer's disease. He was not involved in her current care, he was not specially trained to assess depression, and Ms. Adkins was not terminally ill.

These issues, although important, deflected discussion from what should have been a prior question, the question brought into focus so sharply by the case detailed in this chapter: May a physician ever ethically assist a patient who wishes to commit suicide? Medical ethics tradition for thousands of years has said "no." The Hippocratic oath says "no." "I will give no deadly medicine to anyone if asked, nor suggest any such counsel." More recently, the American College of Physicians *Ethics Manual* (1) has said "no." "Although a patient may refuse a medical intervention and the physician may comply with this refusal, the physician must never intentionally and directly cause death or assist a patient to commit suicide." The American Medical Association says "no." "In assisted suicide . . . the primary purpose of the treatment is to cause death. And that purpose has no role in the professional responsibilities of the physician" (2).

A distinguished panel of physicians, however, recently concluded that "it is not immoral for a physician to assist in the rational suicide of a terminally ill person" (3). Advances in medical technology and compelling cases such as that of Dr. Jones and Ms. Washington require us to look anew at these issues. Withholding or withdrawing life-sustaining treatment, physician-assisted suicide, and active euthanasia form a spectrum of issues in end-of-life decision making. Much has been said about the distinctions between euthanasia and forgoing life-sustaining treatment. This commentary focuses on the issue of physician-assisted suicide.

Conflicting "Goods"

There have always been people who want medicine—through assisted suicide or euthanasia—to help bring about their deaths. Medicine's ability to prolong the dying process in certain circumstances has increased, as has its ability to relieve pain. Not all patients, however, have access to appropriate pain management and supportive care, which may lead some to see suicide as their only option. Good hospice-type care should be a high priority for all patients. Although most patients who do receive quality terminal care find that it meets their needs, a few, like Ms. Washington, want more control.

The "noes" listed earlier in this commentary reflect the fundamental tenet of medicine that physicians be and be seen as healers and comforters, not as agents of death. When physicians cannot heal, however, should life always be sustained? For example, many physicians agree that withdrawing life support from a patient in a persistent vegetative state, once the diagnosis is confirmed, is not unethical when that decision is based on patient wishes.

Is there, as has traditionally been thought, a clear distinction between omitting care at a patient's request that may or may not result in death and actively and intentionally causing (or assisting to cause) death, or between giving someone the means to end his or her own life and directly ending a life? The preservation of life, restoration of health, relief of suffering, and respect for patient autonomy—these four "goods" sometimes conflict. How should they be balanced?

In this case, Dr. Jones wants nothing more than to do what is best for a terminally ill patient for whom he has cared for 20 years. He fears the possibility of a botched suicide attempt. Ms. Washington, knowing she does not have much time, has a clear idea of how she wants to live the remainder of her life. Ms. Washington and Dr. Jones were ultimately able to discuss her views and wishes openly.

In deciding to comply with his patient's wishes, Dr. Jones is doing what he believes will relieve her current and anticipated suffering. In addition, he might say he looked to the principle of patient autonomy as his guide in determining to honor Ms. Washington's request. Ms. Washington had no interest in testing further modern medicine's ability to relieve pain and understood that her strength could not be restored. She foresaw what she believed would soon be a life of increased pain, dependence, and disability.

Sanctity of Life

Physicians are charged to "do no harm." Is there something objectively harmful, or harmful in the eyes of society, about assisting suicide? Ms. Washington maintains that harm will only come to her if Dr. Jones does not help her to live out her remaining time with the peace of mind she will have knowing she can choose death. She is appealing to Dr. Jones to relieve suffering as she defines it. Can harm be done when a person does not acknowledge or recognize it?

Under a "sanctity of human life" argument, the answer would be "yes." Sanctity of life, whether based on religion or on the belief that it is the foundation for social order, dictates that life is sacred and should not be taken. But what about exceptions to the rule? Should physician-assisted suicide ever be such an exception?

"Slippery Slopes" and Other Arguments

Those opposing physician-assisted suicide argue further that the potential consequences of such a practice could have additional

adverse effects on health care: "The dedication of the medical profession to the welfare of patients and to the promotion of their
health might be seriously undermined in the eyes of the public and
of patients by the complicity of physicians in the death of the very
ill" (4). Providing suicide assistance could also compromise patient
trust in physicians (2).

Like "slippery slope" arguments, however, these positions do not
address whether it is ever ethical for physicians to provide suicide
assistance so much as they call attention to the need for rigorous
procedures to safeguard patient rights if assistance was to be sanc-
tioned. Even if in an individual case—for example, assisting the suicide of a thoughtful, emotionally prepared, terminally ill patient
such as Ms. Washington—this practice might seem benevolent, what
would be the social consequences of its acceptance? Would patients
come to feel they have a duty to die? Would more active and less
voluntary forms of euthanasia become acceptable? What about the
risks for error and opportunities for abuse?

These questions are certainly legitimate, but they might be satisfactorily addressed by carefully constructed procedures and some
kind of oversight of the assisted suicide process. The primary question is whether there are circumstances under which it would be ethical for a physician to provide assistance for suicide.

More Unanswered Questions

More questions remain unanswered: Are some patients requesting
assisted suicide because they fear that they will not be allowed to
refuse life support when the time comes? Conversely, would
demands for assisted suicide create a backlash that would make it
more difficult to withhold or withdraw life-sustaining treatment? If
assisted suicide were to become accepted, would physicians have
less incentive to optimize supportive care?

Public interest in the issue of physician-assisted suicide is deep
and pervasive. Opinion polls suggest that approximately equal
numbers favor and oppose it. Clearly, both the medical profession
and society need to continue to discuss the topic and to try to agree
on public and professional policy.

In the meantime, physicians cannot be compelled to assist a suicide, and in considering or acting on these issues, physicians should remember that what they consider ethical may conflict with criminal or civil law, which varies from state to state. Physicians may wish to consult local counsel before taking action that may have legal consequences for themselves, their patients, and their patients' families.

The Future

The practice of medicine has implications that reach far beyond the examination room. The Hippocratic precept of "first, do no harm" today involves harm done to the patient's rights as well as to his or her welfare. Respect for patient autonomy, a hallmark of modern biomedical ethics, dictates that physicians uphold the informed treatment decisions of competent patients. But the medical profession's ethical integrity and obligations to society are threatened when a patient requests physician assistance to commit suicide.

Perhaps what is driving the renewed debate about physician-assisted suicide is the rise of patient autonomy seen in the treatment refusal context. The issue is settled that adult patients (or their surrogates) retain authority for decision making about health care. But how to define the range of patient decisions with which physicians should comply and whether requests for physician-assisted suicide fit into that range are unresolved issues.

Should physician-assisted suicide be permissible under certain circumstances, the next step beyond the withdrawal of feeding tubes and respirators? Or should it be forbidden under all circumstances? The medical profession and society need to decide.

REFERENCES

1. American College of Physicians. American College of Physicians Ethics Manual. Second edition. Ann Intern Med. 1989;111:327-35.
2. Orentlicher D. Physician participation in assisted suicide. JAMA. 1989;262:1844-5.
3. Wanzer SH, Federman DD, Adelstein SJ, Cassel CK, Cassem EH, Cranford RE, et al. The physician's responsibility toward hopelessly ill patients: a second look. N Engl J Med. 1989;320:844-9.

4. Jonsen AR, Siegler M, Winslade WJ. Clinical Ethics. New York: Macmillan; 1986.

ANNOTATED BIBLIOGRAPHY

American Medical Association Council on Ethical and Judicial Affairs. Decisions near the end of life. JAMA. 1992;267:2229-33.

Defines euthanasia, physician-assisted suicide, and the withholding and withdrawing of life-sustaining treatment; discusses these issues in an ethical context; and concludes that physicians must respect competent patients' decisions to refuse life-sustaining treatment and must relieve pain and suffering and promote the dignity of patients, but should not perform euthanasia or participate in assisted suicide.

Brody H. Assisted death—a compassionate response to a medical failure. N Engl J Med. 1992;327:1384-8.

Brody favors physician assistance with suicide under certain circumstances as, the author maintains, appropriate medical practice and a way to re-establish patient trust in the compassion of physicians.

Dying well? A colloquy on euthanasia and assisted suicide. Hastings Cent Rep. 1992;22:6-55.

A collection of eight articles that includes international perspectives and a provocative piece by Daniel Callahan, "When Self-Determination Runs Amok."

Pellegrino ED. Doctors must not kill. J Clin Ethics. 1992;3:95-102; and Compassion needs reason too. JAMA. 1993;270:874-5.

Perhaps among the most eloquent considerations of why physicians should not participate in assisted suicide or euthanasia by one of the founders of modern bioethics.

Quill TE, Cassel CK, Meier DE. Care for the hopelessly ill: proposed clinical criteria for physician-assisted suicide. N Engl J Med. 1992;327:1380-4.

Three physicians propose clinical standards for when and how to comply with patient requests for physician-assisted suicide.

Special supplement on physician-assisted suicide. Hastings Cent Rep. 1995;25:8-25, 36-43.

A collection of articles on medical assistance with death, including current thinking on professional integrity and physician-assisted suicide, the marketing of so-called "death with dignity," hospice care, and more.

Wanzer SH, Adelstein SJ, Cranford RE, Federman DD, Hook E, Moertel CG, et al. The physician's responsibility toward hopelessly ill patients. N Engl J Med. 1984;310:955-9; and Wanzer SH, Federman DD, Adelstein SJ, Cassel

CK, Cassem EH, Cranford RE, et al. The physician's responsibility toward hopelessly ill patients: a second look. N Engl J Med. 1989;320:844-9.

> Physician experts convened by the then Society for the Right to Die (now Choice in Dying) call for flexible care in the treatment of the dying and assert that "it is not immoral for a physician to assist in the rational suicide of a terminally ill person."

3

Physician-Assisted Suicide Revisited: Comfort and Care at the End of Life

Case History and Commentary by SUSAN W. TOLLE, MD, FACP, **and** LOIS SNYDER, JD

CASE HISTORY

Mr. Jensen is a 50-year-old man with colon cancer that has metastasized to the liver. He is at home under the care of his long-time general internist, Sally Jones. Mr. Jensen was diagnosed with cancer in October when a workup for hematochezia showed a mass of 15 cm.

In November, he had a sigmoid-colectomy, and liver nodules were found. A liver biopsy was done, and the results were positive for metastatic adenocarcinoma. After surgery, the patient remained in relatively good health at home for several months. In

Continued

December, he completed a power-of-attorney for health care that appointed his wife as his surrogate decision maker should he become unable to make decisions for himself. He repeatedly expressed to Dr. Jones his strong conviction that he wished to live and fight the disease as long as there was hope for a relatively good quality of life. But when hope was gone, he wanted his life to end; he did not want a drawn-out death like his sister had recently experienced after she was diagnosed with breast cancer. His attitude was generally upbeat, and his wife and two grown sons were close and supportive.

At an office visit in late January, Mr. Jensen is clearly becoming weaker, and oral morphine is no longer fully controlling his pain. Dr. Jones examines him and talks with him and his wife about enrolling in a home hospice program. He agrees and is soon titrated on a self-administered morphine pump to 5 mg/h. His appetite is poor, but he is physically comfortable.

Dr. Jones remains in close contact and receives frequent calls from Mr. Jensen's hospice nurses. Dr. Jones knows that a decision will need to be made in the next few weeks about possible diverting surgery for Mr. Jensen's partial bowel obstruction and the placement of stents for his progressive renal failure. Possible treatment options are discussed with Mr. Jensen. He no longer wants anything done to extend his life—he does not want CPR, does not want to return to the hospital, and does not want surgery. His pain is adequately controlled on 25 mg/h of morphine, but he hates becoming weak and dependent. He asks Dr. Jones to increase the morphine concentration in his self-administered pump so he can take his own life by opening the pump wide (with the current concentration and his poor renal function, fluid overload might precede respiratory suppression). Because of his partial bowel obstruction, he often vomits his medications and does not think he could kill himself with pills. He begs Dr. Jones to order a stronger solution of morphine. His family is aware of his request, and his sons support him in taking this action. His wife is struggling with the request. She is fatigued and remains torn between not wanting him to suffer and not wanting to hasten his death. The hospice nurse believes Mr. Jensen can be kept comfortable with continued good hospice care and finds assisted suicide morally objectionable. Mr. Jensen continues to request assisted suicide. What should Dr. Jones do?

———=▷·◇·◁=———

COMMENTARY

The Patient and His Request

In the second edition of its *Ethics Manual*, the American College of Physicians said an unconditional "no" to assisted suicide, stating that "although a patient may refuse a medical intervention and the physician may comply with this refusal, the physician must never intentionally and directly cause death or assist a patient to commit suicide" (1). Another case study in this book examines the arguments for and against physician-assisted suicide (*see* Chapter 2).

Both society and the College have continued, however, to probe this issue, and in the third edition of the *Ethics Manual*, the College acknowledged that there are difficult situations: "Open conversations between terminally ill patients and their physicians about patient needs and values are essential, even when those conversations include a patient's request for assisted suicide. In most cases, the patient will withdraw the request when pain management, depression, and other concerns have been addressed. But occasionally the issue of physician-assisted suicide needs to be explored in depth" (2). Is Mr. Jensen's case one of those difficult situations? Dissatisfaction with certain aspects of end-of-life care has been evident in public opinion polls and might also have contributed to the approval of, for example, the physician-assisted suicide referendum in Oregon in 1994. Are patient concerns and the right issues being addressed? Are they being addressed here?

The Physician and Patient: Open Communication

What should Dr. Jones do? Are her initial responses contingent on her personal values, professional code, or state laws on assisted suicide, or on a combination of these factors? Are there initial steps all health care providers should take regardless of their views about assisted suicide?

The American Medical Association suggests that "requests for physician-assisted suicide should be a signal to physicians that the patient's needs are unmet, and further evaluation to identify the elements contributing to the patient's suffering is necessary" (3). There is general agreement that the initial response to a request for assisted suicide should be further conversation. This process should begin with an in-depth determination of the patient's unmet needs, fears, suffering, social circumstances, and pain.

Open dialogue frequently yields information about unmet needs. Mr. Jensen may fear a time when his pain will not be controlled. He may fear abandonment. He may be depressed. He may be concerned about his fatigued wife and the burden he perceives he is placing on her. He may feel alone and scared, having not yet thoroughly discussed his wishes and needs. Often through discussions and the interventions of a multidisciplinary team, the patient's suffering will be satisfactorily ameliorated.

The Physician's Obligation: Pain Relief and Symptom Control

Pain relief (4, 5) must be a high priority of medicine, as long as this is what the patient wishes (2). Similarly, the diagnosis and treatment of depression must be given more, and more effective, emphasis in the care of the dying.

Palliative care, the management of pain and symptoms caused by severe illness, includes pain medications and other measures to relieve suffering, such as counseling and support. However, there are barriers to effective palliative care. The gradual increase of pain medication for terminal illness to levels that relieve pain is ethically sound—even if a side effect is to shorten life (2). Some physicians may inappropriately withhold or delay narcotics, fearing that patients will develop a tolerance for them or become addicted to them or that these drugs will hasten death through respiratory suppression (2). Many hospice proponents maintain and are making efforts to persuade the public and physicians that few patients require high doses of pain medication and that even these patients do not become addicted (6). Medicine can benefit from hospice expertise.

Some physicians may not be experienced in methods of pain assessment and control or with interdisciplinary approaches to palliative care. Some pharmacy practices and procedures may also provide obstacles (7). Palliative care experts maintain that pain can be alleviated in all but the rarest of cases (7). Better training and continuing education for health professionals, practice guidelines, patient and public education materials, and changes in pharmacy practices can help make that belief a reality.

Others and Other Issues

In May 1995, the Northern Territory of Australia became the first place in the world to legalize euthanasia. In the Netherlands, euthanasia is not legal, although if established protocols are followed, there is agreement not to prosecute. In the United States, euthanasia is illegal in every state. No state specifically allows assisted suicide. Oregon, however, by popular vote, endorsed physician-assisted suicide in a November 1994 referendum, although a legal injunction presently bars implementation of that measure.

Even if legal prohibitions are lifted, many health professionals and professional societies oppose assisted suicide. Some health care providers find assisting a patient with suicide morally acceptable when all other modalities have been explored and have failed. The number of people who embrace either belief probably varies by jurisdiction. In Washington, a recent survey suggested that health care professionals are evenly split on this issue, similar to the Oregon population (8). Because of general divergence of opinion, members of any health care team may differ on this subject.

In Mr. Jensen's case, the hospice nurse believes that he can and should be kept comfortable and finds assisted suicide objectionable. Even if legal and professional prohibitions are lifted, the expression of moral conscience of each health care provider should be respected. Dr. Jones has an obligation to ensure that she does not coerce or involve the participation of others in an act they find morally reprehensible. Likewise, consideration should be given to the potential burden placed on family members. Mr. Jensen's wife is not decided on the issue, and her current and long-term emotional needs must be considered.

The American College of Physicians continues to probe the issue of physician-assisted suicide. The decision to legalize this practice rests with society and not solely with the medical profession. Each case, however, deserves a respectful hearing and an active effort by the physician to elicit the concerns that led to the patient's request for suicide assistance and to alleviate the patient's distress.

A blanket condemnation of physician-assisted suicide with nothing more misses an opportunity to improve care for dying persons. Physicians have an obligation to understand the stimulus behind the patient's request and to explore with the patient his or her fear, isolation, suffering, depression, pain, and family and economic concerns. Society has an unfulfilled obligation to ensure access to hospice-type resources for all dying persons. The American College of Physicians continues to encourage open conversation, the enhancement of pain relief and symptom control for the dying, and respect for the consciences of all health care providers as we continue to examine the issue of physician-assisted suicide. We affirm a professional ethic that improves the care of patients and families facing these issues.

REFERENCES

1. American College of Physicians. American College of Physicians Ethics Manual. Second edition. Ann Intern Med. 1989;111:245-52, 327-35.
2. American College of Physicians Ethics Manual. Third edition. Ann Intern Med. 1992;117:947-60.
3. American Medical Association. Council on Ethics and Judicial Affairs. Code of Medical Ethics: Reports, vol. V, no. 2. Chicago: American Medical Association; 1994.
4. Agency for Health Care Policy and Research. Management of Cancer Pain. Rockville, Maryland: U.S. Department of Health and Human Services, Public Health Service, Agency for Health Care Policy and Research; 1994. AHCPR publication no. 94-0592.

5. Buchan ML, Tolle SW. Pain relief for dying persons: dealing with physicians' fears and concerns. J Clin Ethics. 1995;6:53-61.
6. Stoddard S. Terminal, but not hopeless. New York Times, August 21, 1991.
7. The New York State Task Force on Life and the Law. When death is sought: assisted suicide and euthanasia in the medical context. New York: New York State Task Force on Life and the Law; 1994.
8. Cohen JS, Fihn SD, Boyko EJ, Jonsen AR, Wood RW. Attitudes toward assisted suicide and euthanasia among physicians in Washington State. N Engl J Med. 1994;331:89-94.

ANNOTATED BIBLIOGRAPHY

Buchan ML, Tolle SW. Pain relief for dying persons: dealing with physicians' fears and concerns. J Clin Ethics. 1995;6:53-61.

> Finds that pain management for terminally ill patients is inadequate. Reviews physician causes of the insufficient use of pain medication and the ethical concepts underlying adequate pain relief.

Bulkin W, Lukashok H. Rx for dying: the case for hospice. N Engl J Med. 1988;318:376-8.

> Describes the growth of the hospice care program, physician obstacles to hospice care, and the role of physicians in hospice.

Conwell Y, Caine ED. Rational suicide and the right to die: reality and myth. N Engl J Med. 1991;325:1100-2.

> Two psychiatrists shed some light on the lack of attention given psychiatric illness in decision making about so-called "rational suicide."

Foley KM. The relationship of pain and symptom management to patient requests for physician-assisted suicide. Journal of Pain and Symptom Management. 1991;6:289-97.

> Maintains that access to expertise in the control of pain and psychological distress and to quality of life must be addressed for patients with cancer.

Miller RJ. Hospice care as an alternative to euthanasia. Law, Medicine and Health Care. 1992;20:127-32.

> Reviews the ethical basis for hospice and considers the question, does hospice care make considerations of euthanasia unnecessary? This author answers "yes."

The New York State Task Force on Life and the Law. When death is sought: assisted suicide and euthanasia in the medical context. New York; New York State Task Force on Life and the Law; 1994.

> Reaffirms prohibitions against physician-assisted suicide and euthanasia and calls for more and better recognition and treatment of depression along with better palliative care.

4

Ethics and Elder Neglect

Case History and Commentary by JANET WEINER, MPH

CASE HISTORY

Cecilia Griffith, age 80, sustained a right hip fracture that was pinned six months ago. Since then, she has been using a wheelchair. Despite physical therapy, she remains unable to walk, even with the aid of a walker.

Arnold Silver, MD, has been the Griffith family's primary care physician for many years. Mr. Griffith died of congestive heart failure about five years ago; subsequently, Ms. Griffith moved in with her son Michael, his wife, and his teenage daughter.

Since her hip fracture, Ms. Griffith has seen Dr. Silver monthly. At this month's visit, he is surprised by her generally disheveled appearance and subdued demeanor. He is also surprised to see Michael because

Continued

Michael's wife usually brings Ms. Griffith to her appointments. Michael explains that he recently lost his job and that his wife has taken a temporary job to keep the family afloat.

On physical examination, Dr. Silver becomes concerned about a few new findings. Ms. Griffith has a decubitus ulcer on her right hip and smells of urine. She denies being incontinent and says she has been feeling the same as usual. She states that she has been staying in bed more because she does not want to go anywhere.

Dr. Silver, having known Ms. Griffith a long time, senses that something has changed in her living situation. He questions her, with Michael out of the room, about the family circumstances. She tells him that Michael is very upset about losing his job and furious that his wife has to go to work. The couple is fighting more than ever.

"It sounds like a stressful situation," Dr. Silver remarks. "How does it affect you?"

"Oh, I try to stay out of everyone's way and not be a burden," Ms. Griffith answers. On close questioning, Dr. Silver finds out that Ms. Griffith has not been to physical therapy in about a month. Michael's wife had been Ms. Griffith's primary caregiver, a role that is now being filled by Michael. Given the physical findings, Dr. Silver suspects that Ms. Griffith is not receiving enough assistance with getting out of bed, reaching the bathroom, and personal hygiene. He worries that continued neglect will have irreparable consequences for Ms. Griffith's health and functional status.

"Is Michael able to give you all the help you need throughout the day?" Dr. Silver asks. "Perhaps you need someone else to help you—would you like me to talk to Michael about it?"

Ms. Griffith becomes agitated and insists that Dr. Silver not bring up the subject with Michael. "He's under so much pressure . . . don't make it worse. I'm fine and I don't need any help."

What should Dr. Silver do?

COMMENTARY

The issue of mistreatment of elderly people was brought into the public view more than a decade ago in the congressional report "Elder Abuse: An Examination of a Hidden Problem" (1). Since then, various state laws, health professionals, and social service agencies have tried to address the problem, with varying degrees of effectiveness. For physicians treating elderly patients, the possibility of abuse or neglect poses both ethical and practical dilemmas. The foregoing case study illustrates some of these dilemmas.

Elder mistreatment covers a spectrum of behaviors, from intentional physical abuse to financial abuse to unintentional neglect. Although the incidence of elder mistreatment is difficult to measure, a congressional subcommittee in 1990 estimated that about 1.5 million people (5% of the nation's elderly population) may be victims each year (2).

All physicians who care for elderly patients should be aware of the signs of elder mistreatment and be able to intervene appropriately. The American Medical Association recently issued guidelines on the diagnosis and treatment of elder abuse that offer physicians guidance on how to recognize and assess mistreatment (3). However, the appropriate course of action for physicians may be clearer in cases of intentional physical violence than in a case such as Ms. Griffith's, which involves unintentional neglect. Dr. Silver, having known the Griffith family for many years, is convinced that Michael does not mean to harm his mother but is probably overwhelmed by his own difficult circumstances and the extent of his mother's care needs. However, the neglect is not benign; it is already having detrimental effects on Ms. Griffith's health, and Dr. Silver must intervene in some way.

This case presents the physician with two fundamental ethical dilemmas: how to balance acting in the patient's best interests with respect for a competent patient's wishes and how to resolve the conflict between the patient's right to confidentiality and the requirements of mandatory reporting laws.

Elderly people have the right to make decisions about their care and their lives. Age alone, in the absence of other factors causing incompetence, should not be a reason to ignore or supersede a patient's wishes. But in this case, Dr. Silver believes that Ms. Griffith's wishes may not be in her best interests. As such, he should handle this situation as he would other types of disagreement between patients and physicians—with extensive and open discussions. He should ensure that Ms. Griffith understands all her options and that her decision is not based on fear or coercion. A dependent elderly person, though competent, may feel intimidated or fear reprisal from her or his caretaker. Dr. Silver should be sensitive to his patient's *perceptions* and how they might affect her decision making. At the same time, Dr. Silver should consider the potential for making the situation worse by possibly leaving his patient open to reprisal or escalation of the mistreatment.

Dr. Silver should determine his next steps using the benchmark of what would be most helpful to Ms. Griffith. His goals should be as follows:

- To help her get the care she needs
  Given the complexity of the medical and psychosocial problems facing the family, referrals should be offered to a comprehensive geriatric center, if available, or to social service agencies that may be able to arrange a visiting nurse or home health or respite services. A home health assessment, either by Dr. Silver or a visiting nurse, may clarify the family situation and pinpoint the specific services that would be most useful.

- To preserve their long-standing physician–patient relationship
  Dr. Silver should find a way to respect his patient's wishes and keep her trust, while still intervening in some fashion. Perhaps Dr. Silver can ask Michael if he knows how to take care of his mother and if he thinks he needs any help or advice. Dr. Silver should avoid blaming the family or patient. It may be best to broach the subject to Michael in terms of his mother's new clinical problem rather than in terms of deficiencies in her care. Dr. Silver could say, "Your mother has developed a new medical problem that needs more care than you can give her yourself . . . let's talk about the options."

- To provide close follow-up and continuing care
  Whether or not additional help is accepted, Dr. Silver should maintain close contact with Ms. Griffith and monitor her condition. He should schedule another appointment soon. As Ms. Griffith's primary care physician, he should be her principal point of contact with the medical system and should facilitate a multidisciplinary approach to her health care.

What should Dr. Silver do if the mistreatment continues (or escalates) and Ms. Griffith's condition worsens? To take the case scenario a step further: In subsequent office visits, Dr. Silver finds that Ms. Griffith may have developed osteomyelitis at the site of her ulcer, and the family remains unwilling to accept any help. At this point, Dr. Silver believes that he needs to take further steps to protect his patient's health and considers whether these circumstances fall into the category of reportable abuse and neglect. Is reporting the situation in his patient's best interests? And if he reports the Griffiths to the state, has he violated his patient's right to confidentiality?

Nearly all states have laws that require various health professionals to report suspected elder abuse and neglect to a state agency (usually Adult Protective Services). Considerable debate exists on the effectiveness of mandatory reporting laws for elder abuse. Conceptually, these laws are similar to child abuse statutes in that they are based on the state's power to protect people who cannot protect themselves. But no such reporting requirement exists in the case of non-elderly, competent adults who have the right to refuse referrals to a state agency. And a recent General Accounting Office study concluded that raising public and professional awareness is a more effective strategy in the identification of cases than are mandatory reporting statutes for elder abuse (4).

Legally, a physician is probably protected from liability if the report is made in good faith. Although little case law exists on the subject, it is also likely that a physician's legal duty to report cases of suspected abuse would supersede physician–patient confidentiality requirements (3). But ethically, the physician must be concerned about how reporting suspected abuse would affect trust and the physician–patient relationship. Practically, the physician must also be concerned about the protective agency's ability to follow up appropriately and the potential for worsening the situation.

Physicians report elder abuse infrequently. One study of physicians in North Carolina documented the perceived barriers to reporting, including confusion about reporting requirements, ignorance of reporting procedures, uncertainty about guarantees of confidentiality, fear of protracted litigation, and cynicism about the state's ability to handle reports (5). Significantly, the study found that physicians who had actually encountered elder abuse had the least confidence in the reporting system.

There is some cause for physician skepticism about the effectiveness of mandatory reporting. State agencies charged with investigating elder abuse and providing services to its victims are often chronically underfunded. According to a 1990 congressional report, states spent annually only $3.80 per elderly resident compared with $45.00 per child on protective services (2). Within admittedly limited state budgets for protective services, less than 4% on average was devoted to services for the elderly.

Dr. Silver must decide whether to report the situation to a state agency. At what point is he legally required to report it? If the situation clearly falls under mandatory reporting requirements, Dr. Silver should report it immediately. If the situation is not clear, Dr. Silver should use his patient's best interests as a standard. Will Ms. Griffith be better off if he reports her case? Can a state agency offer services that will improve the situation for both the patient and family? Dr. Silver's decision should be informed by an accurate understanding of state law and a knowledge of the process that begins with a report of suspected elder mistreatment. Apart from reporting issues, Dr. Silver should maintain close contact with the family and continue to provide ongoing medical care. He should creatively use resources such as visiting nurses and respite care, and if unsuccessful, he should help the patient explore alternative living situations to improve her condition.

REFERENCES

1. Select Committee on Aging, U.S. House of Representatives. Elder Abuse: An Examination of a Hidden Problem. Committee publication no. 97-277, April 1981.
2. Select Committee on Aging, U.S. House of Representatives. Elder Abuse: A Decade of Shame and Inaction. Committee publication no. 101-752, April 1990.
3. American Medical Association. Diagnostic and Treatment Guidelines on Elder Abuse and Neglect. Chicago: American Medical Association; 1993.
4. U.S. General Accounting Office. Elder Abuse: Effectiveness of Reporting Laws and Other Factors. Washington, D.C.: General Accounting Office; 1991.
5. Daniels RS, Baumhover LA, Clark-Daniels CL. Physicians' mandatory reporting of elder abuse. Gerontologist. 1989;29:321-7.

ANNOTATED BIBLIOGRAPHY

American Medical Association Council on Ethical and Judicial Affairs. Physicians and family violence: ethical considerations. JAMA. 1992;267:3190-3.

> Reviews the ethical duty to diagnose and treat family violence based on the principles of beneficence and non-maleficence, the barriers to intervention, confidentiality, and informed consent. Concludes with recommendations for intervention.

Cammer Paris BE, Meier DE, Goldstein T, Weiss M, Fein ED. Elder abuse and neglect: how to recognize warning signs and intervene. Geriatrics. 1995;50:47-53.

> Discusses risk factors and the signs of elder abuse and neglect.

Daniels RS, Baumhover LA, Clark-Daniels CL. Physicians' mandatory reporting of elder abuse. Gerontologist. 1989;29:321-7.

> Physicians who were surveyed were concerned about their competence to diagnose abuse, uncertain about reporting laws, and reluctant to report abuse.

Jecker NS. Privacy beliefs and the violent family: extending the ethical argument for physician intervention. JAMA. 1993;269:776-80.

> Asserts that family privacy concerns make physicians reluctant to respond to domestic violence. Calls for analysis of the physician's ethical duties that includes the principle of justice to encourage intervention.

Lachs MS, Pillemer K. Abuse and neglect of elderly persons. N Engl J Med. 1995;332:437-43.

> Defines abuse, its prevalence and risk factors for the elderly, clinical evaluation, and management and reporting requirements.

PART II

The Patient and Physician: Non-clinical Dimensions of the Relationship

Poking and prodding, tests and prescriptions, and other clinical aspects of direct provision of health care are not the only aspects of the patient–physician relationship. The physician's duties and the patient's appropriate expectations extend beyond the laying on of hands, which is itself a problem if not done for clinical reasons.

Included in this section is a diverse sampling of non-clinical issues affecting the patient–physician relationship: patient demands for particular care in the form of referral requests (Chapter 5) and in the refusal to see a recommended specialist (Chapter 6); what to do about and how to discuss the discovery of a physician's mistake made in the course of care (Chapter 7); and sexual contact between physician and patient (Chapter 8).

5

Referrals and Patient Wishes

Case History and Commentary by LOIS SNYDER, JD

CASE HISTORY

Internist Linda Curtis has been caring for Jack Green, age 48, and his wife Betty for two years, since the retirement of her partner Dr. Smith. The Greens were Dr. Smith's patients for 18 years. Mr. Green is a small-business owner. He has never been seriously ill but is seeing his wife through a long illness with cancer. He seems depressed at a routine cholesterol level check but, despite Dr. Curtis' attempts, is unwilling to talk. He does say that he has not felt like himself lately, noting headaches, allergies, knee pain from an old jogging injury, and a rash on his face and elbows. "I need to feel better quick," he says. "I'd like to see a neurolo-

Continued

35

gist, orthopedic surgeon, and dermatologist. Who do you recommend?"

"Slow down," responds Dr. Curtis. "Let's see if I can't help you first." Mr. Green gets upset. "I really want these problems resolved now—I can't afford to feel under the weather what with Betty sick. And I haven't been able to run very far lately." Running is Mr. Green's passion and his primary exercise and stress relief technique.

After the exam, Dr. Curtis concludes that Mr. Green's problems do not warrant specialist intervention—at least not yet. She wonders if some of these problems are related to the pressure Mr. Green is under and to the physical demands of caring for his wife. She tries again to get him to talk, without success.

"Okay. I'd like to start you on steroid cream for your psoriasis and Chlor-Trimeton for the allergies. The headaches are likely related to the allergies and to stress. Your joint is stable, but I will talk to an orthopedic surgeon and determine whether a consultation is warranted. Let's see how it goes. I'd like you to come back next week." Dr. Curtis is not convinced of the need for an orthopedist either but feels pressured by Mr. Green's requests.

Dr. Curtis wants to talk further, but Mr. Green cuts her off. "If you won't get me the help I need, I'll have to get it myself." An unhappy Mr. Green leaves, but he does take his prescription and schedules a follow-up appointment.

Dr. Curtis talks to orthopedic surgeon Sam Jackson, who after hearing the history and evaluation, concurs that Dr. Curtis is on the appropriate course. Dr. Curtis makes a note to check Mr. Green's insurance coverage. She has just started participating in HealthE, an IPA-model HMO, and she is learning its procedures. If Mr. Green is with HealthE, he will need written referrals to specialists for that care to be covered.

Mr. Green returns for his follow-up visit. His symptoms are beginning to improve but not enough to satisfy him. On further discussion, he agrees that he does not really need to see a neurologist or dermatologist but remains emphatic about wanting to see an orthopedist. "Where's Dr. Smith when I need him? He would have recommended specialists to me at the last visit," says Mr. Green.

Dr. Curtis has determined that Mr. Green is a fee-for-service patient, so no written referral is needed. But Mr. Green mentions that as part of the yearly review of benefits at his company, he is considering switching coverage for his family and his employees to an HMO, perhaps HealthE. "Would you be referring me if I had different coverage?" he asks. He says he is going to call his insurer to complain. How should Dr. Curtis handle this?

———◆———

COMMENTARY

When is a consultation warranted? The third edition of the American College of Physicians *Ethics Manual* states, "Physicians should obtain consultation when they feel a need for assistance in caring for the patient or when it is requested by the patient" (1). Does this mean referrals should be made on demand? The short answer is "no."

Referrals should be made when they are in the patient's best interest. Determining what is in the patient's best interest is a matter of professional judgment and medical indication, not a function of patient pressure, peer or institutional pressures about the cost of care, what type of insurance the patient may have, or the physician's payment arrangement (1; *see also* Chapter 14). But with an insistent patient, standing firm on clinical judgment might be easier said than done.

"The welfare of the patient is always paramount in the consultation process," as it is in all aspects of the physician–patient relationship, states the *Ethics Manual* (1). The conflict here is in who is defining that welfare and how—the patient wants immediate intervention for what he sees as a problem requiring a specialist, while Dr. Curtis believes the issue for now is evaluation, which she is competent to handle. However, the physician is in the position to determine what is medically indicated. Managed care policies, for example, often place the primary care physician in the role of "gatekeeper" and thus potentially limit the patient's freedom of choice.

Indeed, all physicians have an obligation to use health resources appropriately and efficiently, avoiding unnecessary tests (including unjustified repetition of tests) and unnecessary consultations. First, the physician must be a patient advocate. But being a patient advocate does not necessarily mean doing everything the patient wants. And the traditional approach to patient advocacy is also being challenged by the need to be conscious of societal and institutional concerns about resource allocation (2).

In Mr. Green's case, Dr. Curtis sees no societal—or institutional—patient conflict. She believes, and the orthopedic surgeon concurs, that she is on the right course in evaluating and following Mr. Green's knee condition. Dr. Curtis' greatest challenge is effectively communicating this fact to Mr. Green. The physician and patient must thoroughly discuss their concerns and expectations. Dr. Curtis may not be able to change Mr. Green's expectations (although she was successful regarding the dermatologist and neurologist), but she is right to try. She should continue to try by informing the patient about her approach to care, the need to allow time for healing, and her discussion with Dr. Jackson.

Physicians should try to help patients develop realistic expectations about medical care. More care is not necessarily better care, and tests carry risk and can result in false-positive results, thereby increasing stress and leading to potential complications. Perhaps for the patient's previous physician, Dr. Smith, being a patient advocate meant doing what the patient wanted and doing more—although nearly 20 years ago there was less "more" to do.

The Greens are fee-for-service patients, which Dr. Curtis did not know at the time of her original recommendation. The payment arrangement was correctly not part of her thinking about a care plan for Mr. Green. Payment arrangements can be a subtle, or not so subtle, influence on clinical judgment. An HMO doctor might take a wait-and-see approach for too long: Under some contractual arrangements with HMOs, for example, physicians agree to a percentage withholding of their fees that is returned only if their referral account for specialist and laboratory services has a surplus at the year's end. Often, bonuses are also given for running a surplus. In the fee-for-service context, a physician could too quickly order, or repeat, a test or make a referral because of the financial incentive to do more and therefore be paid more (3, 4; *see also* Chapter 14).

Mr. Green has said he is considering changing coverage. Under the rules of HealthE, patients need a written referral from the primary care physician for specialist care to be covered. Dr. Curtis needs to discuss this fact with the patient and encourage him to talk to HealthE about the details of coverage, so that he understands the rationale behind preauthorized referrals and other terms of coverage. Such an understanding is essential if Mr. Green is to make an informed choice among insurance plans.

Mr. Green has also said that he will complain to his current insurer, which he is free to do. He may even start to talk about legal action. But the practice and documentation of medically appropriate care are the best defenses to challenges about that care, legal or otherwise.

If after several weeks of conservative management, Mr. Green is not better, or if evidence exists of a ligament injury or increased swelling, Dr. Curtis will want to rethink her position on referral. But for now, referral seems unnecessary and not beneficial to the patient.

If Mr. Green remains adamant about seeing an orthopedist, he will likely find one on his own. If on a subsequent visit Mr. Green persists in wanting names, then Dr. Curtis should at that point give him names of physicians she usually recommends. If he switches to HealthE, she should explain to Mr. Green that physician visits, tests, and treatment without a referral would be at his expense. Regardless of the insurance coverage, Dr. Curtis should tell Mr. Green that she believes a referral is not medically indicated or in his best interest at this time.

REFERENCES

1. American College of Physicians. American College of Physicians Ethics Manual. Third edition. Ann Intern Med. 1992;117:947-60.
2. Wolf SM. Health care reform and the future of physician ethics. Hastings Center Report. 1994;24:28-41.

3. Hillman AL. Health maintenance organizations, financial incentives and physicians' judgments. Ann Intern Med. 1990;112:891-3.
4. Rodwin MA. Medicine, Money, and Morals: Physicians' Conflicts of Interest. New York: Oxford University Press; 1993.

ANNOTATED BIBLIOGRAPHY

Miles SH. Informed demand for "non-beneficial" medical treatment. N Engl J Med. 1991;325:512-5.

Analyzes the Helga Wanglie case and a family's fight to continue life-sustaining treatment against medical advice. Argues that patient desires do not create an entitlement to inappropriate care.

Wolf SM. Health care reform and the future of physician ethics. Hastings Center Report. 1994;24:28-41.

Discusses ethical tensions inherent in various health care delivery models and in efforts at cost consciousness and containment; analyzes proposals for clarifying physician obligations and proposes the development of a new ethics of institutions.

6

Patient Prejudice

Case History and Commentary by **Errol D. Crook, MD, and Lois Snyder, JD**

CASE HISTORY

Mr. Smith is a 60-year-old white man who presents to his internist, Dr. Johnson, with intermittent chest pain that he says he has had for several days. Dr. Johnson has cared for Mr. Smith for many years and knows that he would not visit a doctor unless he was having significant problems. His pain has been occurring during lower and lower levels of physical activity and now sometimes occurs when he is resting. After examining Mr. Smith and doing an electrocardiogram, Dr. Johnson is concerned about the possibility of unstable angina and decides that Mr. Smith

Continued

needs to be hospitalized for further evaluation and treatment.

Dr. Johnson admits Mr. Smith to the intensive care unit. He asks Dr. Natal, a board-certified cardiologist, to see Mr. Smith. Dr. Johnson and his partner have referred many of their cardiac patients to Dr. Natal for several years and believe him to be thorough and to have a good bedside manner with patients. All of their patients have seemed happy with Dr. Natal's care.

Dr. Natal sees Mr. Smith that afternoon. As the doctor is taking his history, Mr. Smith starts to experience typical anginal chest pain associated with some mild electrocardiographic changes. Dr. Natal is able to relieve Mr. Smith's pain with sublingual nitroglycerin and intravenous antianginal agents, but he thinks that cardiac catheterization is warranted. He discusses the situation with Mr. Smith and makes plans to perform the procedure in the morning. Mr. Smith is hesitant but agrees to have the procedure done if Dr. Johnson is in favor of it. The patient has two more episodes of chest pain that afternoon.

Dr. Johnson visits Mr. Smith later, after discussing his care with Dr. Natal. Dr. Johnson tells Mr. Smith that he agrees the catheterization is needed. Mr. Smith responds, "I know that I need something done, but will you be there?" As Dr. Johnson is explaining that he will not be present during the procedure, he senses that Mr. Smith is becoming upset. He asks what is wrong.

"Dr. Johnson," Mr. Smith starts hesitantly, "I would rather have another cardiologist." Dr. Johnson replies that Dr. Natal is very good and has seen many of his patients. Mr. Smith is still not satisfied. After further discussion that includes questions about Dr. Natal's medical training and heritage, it becomes obvious that Mr. Smith is not comfortable with a "foreign doctor."

Dr. Johnson is quite surprised. He respectfully attempts to convince Mr. Smith that Dr. Natal has his full support and utmost confidence. He reiterates, "Dr. Natal is very well trained and is one of the most respected cardiologists in the area." Mr. Smith remains steadfast in his desire for another cardiologist.

What should Dr. Johnson do? Should he continue in his efforts to convince Mr. Smith of Dr. Natal's qualifications? Should he inform Dr. Natal that Mr. Smith wants a different doctor? Should he suggest that Mr. Smith tell Dr. Natal himself

⎯⎯⎯⟫•◇•⟪⎯⎯⎯

COMMENTARY

Establishing a good physician–patient relationship is primary to the practice of medicine. Maintaining such a relationship often requires the handling of delicate and complex issues. No longer is this relationship paternalistic, with the physician acting as the sole decision maker; instead, the physician–patient relationship has become a partnership, with shared decision making. Differences in culture, religion, or certain ideological beliefs may strain and, in some cases, sever the union. This case shows how perceived differences can threaten a physician–patient relationship and affect patient care.

Discrimination of any kind toward patients or colleagues has no place in medicine. A physician may not discriminate against a class or category of patients (1). Patients are obviously not bound by a professional code of conduct as are physicians. They have their own aims and values, which play a major role in their care.

Dr. Johnson is faced with a serious dilemma. What he believes is best for the patient, best for a peer, and consonant with his ideas of right and wrong appear to be a potential threat to his patient's confidence in him. And, as the American College of Physicians *Ethics Manual* states, "The patient's welfare and best interests must be the physician's main concern. . . . In all instances, the physician must help maintain the dignity of the person and respect the uniqueness of each person" (1). Dr. Johnson's actions must be guided by these principles.

His primary concern has to be for Mr. Smith, his patient of many years. Dr. Johnson had his patient's best interest in mind when he referred him to Dr. Natal. This reasoning must be respectfully communicated (3), and Dr. Johnson should attempt to convince Mr. Smith of Dr. Natal's medical expertise. Dr. Johnson should also keep Mr. Smith well informed about the consequences of his decision. If, for instance, Dr. Natal were the only cardiologist in the area, Mr. Smith would have to transfer to another facility to avoid being under Dr. Natal's care.

The reasons for Mr. Smith's request should be examined. Dr. Johnson may be uncomfortable with having to elicit from the patient what the problem is, but he needs to do so both to resolve this situation and to inform his decisions about subsequent referrals. When female patients request female physicians, many physicians will try to comply without question. Sometimes a patient will request a physician with whom he has had a previous relationship or one who was recommended by a family member or an older, "more experienced" doctor. In other circumstances, communications barriers might interfere with the provision of care. But in this case, Dr. Natal has no English-language problems, and although physician communication styles and personalities can result in different comfort levels for patients, Dr. Johnson knows Dr. Natal to have generally good communication skills and an excellent bedside manner.

The distinction between patient preferences and discrimination can sometimes be cloudy, although not in this case. Mr. Smith's request is based on his biases against people who do not share his cultural background, and the request should be challenged, but in a manner that does not undermine the patient's condition or the physician–patient relationship. Although the reasons that Mr. Smith has asked for another cardiologist may seem discriminatory, it is his prerogative to do so. Dr. Johnson is correct to try to educate him, but ultimately, the doctor need not agree with or understand Mr. Smith's wishes. However, those wishes must be respected because the patient has the right to choose. Dr. Johnson must recognize that each patient comes into the relationship with his or her own set of values and desires. If Dr. Johnson believes that Dr. Natal is being unfairly discriminated against and does not want to be involved, he has the option of recommending a physician to take his place and withdrawing from the case.

Clearly, physicians are not immune from biases against certain groups. The biases that exist in American culture are also found in American medicine. Such discrimination persists despite laws prohibiting it in many areas of public life. A physician like Dr. Natal may experience even more discrimination because of what is perceived by some to be an "unusual" name, a particular complexion, a different manner of dress, or an accent. Many international medical graduates have suffered from discrimination. Not only have they experienced bias from patients but from hospitals, training programs, and other physicians as well (3). Where a doctor's medical training occurs is not the only determinant in discrimination: Many U.S.-trained physicians of foreign birth or ancestry have experienced the same problems. They often find it difficult to get referrals and in some cases to obtain privileges.

What should Dr. Johnson do to maintain his strong professional relationship with Dr. Natal? Although Dr. Johnson's primary obligation is to his patient, he also has a professional obligation to his colleague. He must not allow this episode, or the chance that similar occurrences may happen, to sway his referral pattern. Dr. Natal's qualifications and abilities as a physician are without question, and past referrals have had excellent results.

It would be inappropriate and potentially damaging to Dr. Johnson's relationship with Mr. Smith for the doctor to insist that the patient tell Dr. Natal about his wishes himself. Is Dr. Johnson then obligated to inform Dr. Natal about this? Physicians should treat not only their patients, but also each other, with respect. Dr. Johnson should assure Dr. Natal that he has his continued support and confidence and that this incident will not change his referral practices in any way.

Because the United States is made up of diverse peoples who sometimes clash, it is important to learn and exercise the skills to solve problems when they arise and to also help patients learn. Many physicians may face problems similar to those faced by Dr. Johnson. As professionals, physicians occupy positions of significant influence. Therefore, they can—and should—move people away from bigotry, not just by their words but by their actions.

REFERENCES

1. American College of Physicians. American College of Physicians Ethics Manual. Third edition. Ann Intern Med. 1992;117:947-60.
2. Brock DW, Wartman SA. When competent patients make irrational choices. N Engl J Med. 1990;322:1595-9.
3. Doyle E. Foreign-born doctors charge discrimination, fight back with grievances, court challenges. ACP Observer. December 1993;13:1, 13-4.

ANNOTATED BIBLIOGRAPHY

Brock DW, Wartman SA. When competent patients make irrational choices. N Engl J Med. 1990;322:1595-9.

> Patients have a right to make unusual treatment decisions if they are competent. Physicians, however, may try to convince patients to reconsider irrational choices. This article distinguishes the unusual from the irrational and discusses the physician and patient role in shared treatment decision making.

7

Disclosure of Errors and the Threat of Malpractice

Commentary by LOIS SNYDER, JD, and TROYEN A. BRENNAN, MD, JD, MPH, FACP
Case History by TROYEN A. BRENNAN, MD, JD, MPH, FACP

CASE HISTORY

Dr. Howard McGregor has been concerned about his busy internal medicine practice. He has contracts with several managed care plans and is now seeing an average of 16 patients per half-day session. As few as three years ago, he was seeing only nine patients per session. Sometimes he wonders if he is adequately following up on tests and procedures.

Today, he is seeing Karen Madner, a 53-year-old woman who has been his patient since she was in her

Continued

late 30s. She had three children and then had a tubal ligation. She is very concerned about breast cancer because her mother and sister were both diagnosed late with and died of breast cancer. They died at age 48 and 40, respectively. She no longer sees an obstetrician-gynecologist, and Dr. McGregor provides her gynecologic care.

Ms. Madner's last visit was approximately 16 months ago. She usually has a yearly follow-up, at which time she has a Pap smear and a mammogram. In reviewing Ms. Madner's record before she comes in, Dr. McGregor is shocked to find that the previous mammogram report (16 months before) suggested an abnormality and called for follow-up in four months. The radiologist's note was fairly explicit about the suspicious nature of the lesion and the need for expedient follow-up. Dr. McGregor has no idea how he could have overlooked this report.

He examines Ms. Madner and finds a palpable lump in the area of the abnormality. At this point, he is anxious and irritated. He questions Ms. Madner about her use of breast self-examination, which she says she does religiously; then he suggests that she should have a mammogram immediately and should also be referred to a surgeon. "What's going on?" she asks. "I had a normal mammogram last time." Ms. Madner is, of course, quite upset as well, but Dr. McGregor is so agitated that he does a poor job of attending to her emotional concerns.

After Ms. Madner leaves, Dr. McGregor has time for reflection. He recalls that Ms. Madner is a single mother who works full time to support her two high-school-aged children. Diagnosis of and treatment for breast cancer could have a significant effect on her ability to continue working. He wonders if she has disability insurance and makes a note to ask her.

Dr. McGregor then calls his senior colleague Dr. Rendler for advice. Dr. Rendler is surprised that Dr. McGregor did not have a more engaging discussion with the patient. Dr. Rendler believes that full disclosure of mistakes with patients is the best course. She explains that she has been in similar situations and has always found that the outcome is best when mistakes are shared honestly with the patient. Patients are less likely to sue if so informed and are better able to cope with the disease.

Dr. McGregor considers what to do next. What should he decide?

⟹◆⟸

COMMENTARY

To err is human. No one is immune. But when physicians err, the stakes obviously can be quite high.

The issue here is not how to eliminate error, which is an unobtainable goal. Nonetheless, the goal of eliminating error clearly influences the culture and world view of medicine. One physician views mistakes as ". . . a crime. . . . There's some anonymous court that's been set up someplace—I mean Osler or God somewhere at Massachusetts General Hospital—and you've been convicted and tried at the same time" (1).

Physicians, perhaps by nature and certainly as a result of their training, often strive to attain perfection in their practice of medicine (2, 3). Lucian Leape, MD, has commented on this phenomenon: "One result is that physicians, not unlike test pilots, come to view an error as a failure of character—you weren't careful enough, you didn't try hard enough" (3). This sensibility often becomes pronounced among residents (*see* Chapter 13).

Perhaps the only people who seem to demand perfection in medicine more than doctors are patients. Patients sometimes have unrealistic expectations about what medicine and their physicians can do for them and unrealistic views about the possibility of error in the provision of health care. This viewpoint, too, influences how physicians handle mistakes. Physicians should keep patients well informed and help them to have reasonable expectations. Patients, however, should be able to expect that their care will be given appropriate attention and follow-up. It is the physician's obligation to do so.

Of course, errors should be prevented, when possible, but some mistakes are inevitable, sometimes as a result of negligence, sometimes not. The potential for error is great in a complicated endeavor like medicine and in complex settings such as hospitals. The Harvard Medical Practice Study randomly sampled 51 New York hospitals and found that among discharged patients, 1% suffered harm because of negligence (4). In another study, patients in intensive care units were found to have been subject to an average of 178 separate "activities" and 1.7 errors per day per patient; 29% of the errors were characterized as potentially serious or fatal (3).

Reflecting on this study, Dr. Leape notes that 1.7 errors per day means a 99% proficiency rate. However, he also notes that a 1% error is much higher than that found acceptable in, for example, dangerous industries such as aviation and nuclear power. He concludes that although physicians, nurses, and pharmacists "probably are among the most careful professionals in our society," they are not proficient at error prevention because "they have a great deal of difficulty in dealing with human error when it does occur" (3). In addition, who was responsible for the mistake may not be immediately apparent, or individuals may deny responsibility (5).

So we come to the issue at hand: how to deal with error while maintaining ethical obligations to the patient and respecting patient rights.

The third edition of the American College of Physicians *Ethics Manual* directs physicians to ". . . disclose to patients information about procedural or judgment errors made in the course of care, if such information significantly affects the care of the patient" (6). The manual goes on to say that "errors do not necessarily constitute improper, negligent, or unethical behavior" (6). But failure to disclose a significant error can be all three.

Dr. McGregor should have a longer discussion with Ms. Madner about the previously overlooked lesion on the mammogram. Ms. Madner has a right to information that significantly affects her care. She also needs to be well informed to make further decisions about her care and to work in partnership with Dr. McGregor. "Effective patient–physician communication can dispel uncertainty and fear and enhance healing and patient satisfaction" (6). Such communication can also help dispel the anger and confusion that often contribute to the filing of malpractice lawsuits.

The threat of legal action is real. Most liability insurers would probably want to be notified very early, either on discovery of the mistake or shortly thereafter. Although the physician might hold himself or herself to a standard of perfection, the legal system does not. Instead, what is required is that the physician practice with reasonable care, that is, as a similarly trained physician would do in similar circumstances.

Apart from potentially preventing legal action, effective communication can help maintain or restore the trust necessary to a good patient–physician relationship. In this instance, Ms. Madner clearly knows or will know soon that something went awry. This error is not undetectable to a layperson. Even if it were, the standard for disclosure is not detectability. The standard is whether or not information about the error will significantly affect the patient's care. To say nothing here is unethical, and that course of action would undermine or ultimately destroy the patient–physician relationship.

Dr. McGregor is right to be very concerned about the potential consequences of the mistake and of disclosure and to give thought to how he will broach the discussion with his patient and what he might say. He might further discuss the situation with Dr. Rendler, while maintaining patient confidentiality, in preparation for his conversation with Ms. Madner. He should also think about changes in his practice or office procedures that would help him avoid such mistakes in the future, for example, a review of his patient load and attention to how lab reports are screened. Acknowledging an error and accepting responsibility for it can be the first steps in improving quality of care. He should, however, talk to the patient sooner rather than later, and her care should not be delayed further.

Dr. McGregor might also benefit from any support Dr. Rendler or other colleagues can provide him. The emotional impact of the mistake process can take a toll on physicians. "The medical profession simply seems to have no place for its mistakes. There is no permission given to talk about errors, no way of venting emotional responses. Indeed, one would almost think that mistakes are in the same category as sins . . . " (2). Physicians should find a place to talk about mistakes; to deal with them and the responses they engender, emotional and otherwise; and to learn from them. And then they should move on.

REFERENCES

1. Christensen JF, Levison W, Dunn PM. The heart of darkness: the impact of perceived mistakes on physicians. J Gen Intern Med. 1992;7:424-31.
2. Hilfiker D. Facing our mistakes. N Engl J Med. 1984;310:118-22.
3. Leape LL. Error in medicine. JAMA. 1994;272:1851-7.
4. Localio AR, Lawthers AG, Brennan TA, Laird NM, Herbert LE, Peterson LM, et al. Relation between malpractice claims and adverse events due to negligence: results of the Harvard Medical Practice Study III. N Engl J Med. 1991;325:245-51.
5. Lo B. Disclosing mistakes. In: Lo B, ed. Resolving Ethical Dilemmas: A Guide for Clinicians. Baltimore: William & Wilkins; 1995:307-13.
6. American College of Physicians. American College of Physicians Ethics Manual. Third edition. Ann Intern Med. 1992;117:947-60.

ANNOTATED BIBLIOGRAPHY

Christensen JF, Levison W, Dunn PM. The heart of darkness: the impact of perceived mistakes on physicians. J Gen Intern Med. 1992;7:424-31.

Physicians were interviewed about previous mistakes and their impact on the physicians' lives and practices. Among the conclusions of the study were that perceived errors caused emotional distress and that sharing this distress with colleagues varied on the basis of competitiveness as a result of medical training. The authors call for more open discussion of mistakes in practice and training.

Hilfiker D. Facing our mistakes. N Engl J Med. 1984;310:118-22.

A physician shares a significant mistake, its effects, and his thoughts on the need for acknowledgment and discussion of errors among peers.

Leape LL. Error in medicine. JAMA. 1994;272:1851-7.

Looks at the potential for error in medicine, at attitudes toward errors and prevention, and at possible changes to hospital systems to prevent or identify errors in a timely fashion.

Leape LL, Bates DW, Cullen DJ, Cooper J, Demonaco HJ, Gullivan T, et al. Systems analysis of adverse drug events. JAMA. 1995;274:35-43.

Identifies and reviews errors in prescribing and administering drugs that result from systems failures, with an eye toward changes to the system to improve drug and patient information.

8

Sex and the Single Physician

Case History and Commentary by JANET WEINER, MPH, **and** SUSAN W. TOLLE, MD, FACP

CASE HISTORY

Leonard Sullivan, MD, age 59, has been one of three general internists in Pumpkin Hills, Wyoming, for the past 30 years. He came to Pumpkin Hills immediately after his residency, married a local woman, and raised two children who are now away at college. Dr. Sullivan's wife died of breast cancer one year ago.

Margaret Dinardo, age 60, has spent her life in Pumpkin Hills and has been a patient of Dr. Sullivan's for nearly 20 years. Her husband died two years ago, and her children are now married with families of their own.

Continued

Ms. Dinardo returns for her yearly visit with Dr. Sullivan. He finds her in continued good health, renews her Feldene prescription for mild osteoarthritis, and schedules her yearly mammogram. Dr. Sullivan reviews the results of his clinical exam, and they talk about general preventive care measures. He notices that he feels uplifted by Ms. Dinardo's presence.

"Enough about me, Leonard," Ms. Dinardo says finally. "How have you been since Diane passed on?"

"It's been difficult, although the children have been a great help," he responds. Ms. Dinardo touches his shoulder, saying, "I know exactly what you mean," and leaves.

About a week later, Ms. Dinardo calls Dr. Sullivan at home and invites him over for dinner. "I bet you don't get many home-cooked meals these days," she says. He accepts the invitation, and they spend the evening talking. Dr. Sullivan tells her about his life now and the trouble he has had coping with his wife's death. In Margaret Dinardo he finds an understanding and compassionate listener, who shares the experiences she has had since losing her spouse. "Thank you, Margaret . . . I feel so much better talking to you," he says.

"Any time, Leonard," she responds. "Call me and maybe we'll catch a movie."

In the next few months, Dr. Sullivan and Ms. Dinardo see each other regularly. They enjoy each other's company and consider their relationship to be an evolution of their long-standing friendship. But Dr. Sullivan begins to notice that he feels romantically inclined toward Ms. Dinardo and wonders if she feels the same way. One evening, Ms. Dinardo says, "Leonard, what is the matter with you? You've been fidgeting since you got here." He blurts out that he feels attracted to her romantically, and she replies, "Well, it's about time! I was beginning to think you were just too old for me!"

They kiss passionately, well into the evening. He reluctantly draws away from her and heads toward the door. "I really should be getting home. I have a busy day tomorrow at the office. Good night, Margaret."

"Oh, well, your duty calls. Good night, Dr. Sullivan," she replies.

He does not sleep at all, feeling strangely disquieted by the word "doctor." All day, he is troubled by Ms. Dinardo's use of "Dr. Sullivan." After a long day at the office, he decides to talk to her about it. "You know, I was always taught that a sexual relationship between a doctor and a patient is wrong," he begins. "If we're going to start something here, maybe you should consider becoming Dr. Voorhees' patient."

Ms. Dinardo reacts with surprise and anger. "Leonard Sullivan, you have been my doctor for 20 years. I trust you—that doesn't just go away because we kissed. How can you even think such a thing?" She refuses to consider seeing another internist. "Listen, we kissed yesterday, and you expect me to give you up as a doctor? You must be kidding!"

What should Dr. Sullivan do?

⟾⬦⬅

COMMENTARY

This case study illustrates some of the subtleties and difficulties inherent in the general prohibition of sex between doctor and patient. The prohibition dates back to at least the Hippocratic Oath, which states, "I will come for the benefit of the sick, remaining free of all intentional injustice, of all mischief and in particular of sexual relations with both male and female persons . . . " (1). Although medical and ethical consensus on this prohibition remains intact, recently publicized abuses have brought renewed public and professional attention to the issue.

The College's *Ethics Manual* is clear on this point: "It is unethical for a physician to become sexually involved with a current patient even if the patient initiates or consents to the advances" (2). Likewise, the American Medical Association concludes that "sexual contact or a romantic relationship with a patient concurrent with the physician–patient relationship is unethical" (1). Both sources also question the wisdom of sexual relationships with former patients. The American Medical Association and American College of Physicians consider it unethical "if the physician uses or exploits trust, knowledge, emotions, or influence derived from the previous professional relationship" (1).

Four arguments form the foundation for a prohibition against sexual contact between physician and patient:

1. The inequality between the parties
   In doctor–patient relationships, patients answer personal questions, reveal sensitive information, and allow the doctor to touch them. This intimacy is one-way; doctors do not ordinarily put themselves in similar positions. True consent by the patient to an intimate relationship is questionable, and initiation of such a relationship is suspect, given this inequality.

2. The inherent vulnerability of the patient
   Most patients who seek care are ill and put great faith in the doctor's opinion and advice. The inequality in knowledge and health status puts patients in a vulnerable and dependent position, one that physicians must never exploit.

3. The possibility of betraying the patient's trust
   The social contract between physicians and patients is based on trust: Patients trust that doctors will keep all information confidential and will only use this information to help them. At some point in an intimate relationship, a doctor could use knowledge gained from the therapeutic relationship out of self-interest or a patient or community might believe exploitation has occurred. A misuse of information undermines trust in the profession as a whole.

4. The conflict with the physician's duty to act in the patient's best interests
   In the therapeutic relationship, patients trust that doctors will keep patients' interests primary. In a sexual relationship, there are competing and sometimes conflicting interests. The two relationships cannot be reconciled.

For these reasons, sex between doctors and current patients is considered unethical. Ethical concerns are mirrored in legal and regulatory sanctions against this practice. The laws of several states consider sexual contact between physicians and patients to be criminal behavior, and such contact is almost universally grounds for action by state licensing boards.

In many ways, the case study detailed here is not typical of sexual misconduct by doctors who abuse their patients. We do not mean to ignore or diminish this reality with the case we have presented. For example, the case of an obstetrician raping a patient under anesthesia or of a psychiatrist having sex with a patient under the guise of therapy is so obviously wrong that the ethics need no explanation. To explore whether the professional ethic holds true in less obvious situations, we have deliberately crafted the most benign, long-standing physician–patient relationship we could imagine.

Despite prohibitions discussed above, investigators have found that 5% to 10% of all psychiatrists report sexual contact with a patient, and these figures likely hold true for other specialists as well (3). Most of this contact appears to clearly exploit the patient within the therapeutic relationship. There are well-documented reports of harm to patients from these relationships, which can have devastating effects on their lives and their capacity to trust other physicians. In these published studies, 85% to 90% of patients consider sexual contact with their physician to have been damaging, although the data may be biased by selective reporting of more negative reactions (1). Female patients (overwhelmingly the objects of such contact) have been reported to experience guilt, severe distrust of their own judgment, and mistrust of both men and physicians.

We turn now to the more difficult type of case, like our Dr. Sullivan's, in which the physician and patient find themselves attracted to one another in a relationship concurrent with, but apart from, the therapeutic relationship. This problem can be particularly difficult in small rural communities, where a large proportion of the community may be the physician's patients.

On the surface, our case lacks many of the aspects that make physician–patient sex so disconcerting: Ms. Dinardo does not seem especially vulnerable because she is not acutely or chronically ill. Dr. Sullivan does not seem to be betraying Ms. Dinardo's trust, and their relationship does not seem unequal. Indeed, they seem to step out of their roles of patient and physician in the social context in which they continue to see each other. Should this kind of situation be considered just a matter of consensual activity between two adults? Does the ethical prohibition apply, and if so, why?

In our case, the dangers are subtle but still present. Twenty years of a therapeutic relationship may have produced a dependence in Ms. Dinardo that Dr. Sullivan does not recognize. Indeed, Dr. Sullivan's willingness to transfer Ms. Dinardo's care to another physician and her extreme objection to being transferred point to a difference in both perception and power. Physicians and patients may view a sexual relationship quite differently and may not share the same understanding of the effect of their ongoing or previous therapeutic relationship.

If Dr. Sullivan tries to maintain a dual relationship, he would violate a fundamental tenet of medical ethics and physician practice— the promise to keep his patient's interests primary. This violation would occur regardless of the outcome of their intimate relationship. In a sexual relationship, Dr. Sullivan necessarily elevates his own interests to at least the same level as his patient's. He begins to act in his own best interest. Perhaps these interests converge with his patient's, and they will live happily ever after. In that case, Dr. Sullivan's objectivity would be colored, and we would recommend that he not continue to take care of Ms. Dinardo for many of the same reasons physicians should not provide ongoing medical care to family members.

There is, however, no guarantee of future happiness. One of the arguments against physician–patient sex is that the relationship might not last forever. Dr. Sullivan and Ms. Dinardo could embark on an intimate relationship that eventually will fall apart. Perhaps the breakup would not be without rancor. In any event, Dr. Sullivan and Ms. Dinardo could probably not continue a trusting doctor–patient relationship, and one or both would want to sever the professional ties. In that scenario, it is clearer that the patient's interests did not remain primary and led to a conflict of interest.

Therefore, in either scenario, it would not be in Ms. Dinardo's best interests to remain as Dr. Sullivan's patient. It would also not be in Dr. Sullivan's best interests. He risks losing his license if he is reported to the state board and risks losing the confidence of his other patients and the community if he becomes intimate with a current patient. Because Dr. Sullivan knows what the ethical considerations and risks are, it is important for him to resolve the issue of transfer of Ms. Dinardo's care to another physician before he and Ms. Dinardo begin an intimate relationship.

Even former patients may continue to feel dependent or vulnerable, and Dr. Sullivan should carefully assess this possibility (consultation with an objective colleague may help). The danger to former patients of a relationship with their psychiatrist has been recognized by criminal or civil laws in several states (4). Most of these laws dictate a one- to two-year interval as an appropriate safeguard against abuse. Of course, internists may not face the same issues of transference and power imbalance as do psychiatrists. The delay necessary to protect a patient will vary with the people involved and the nature, extent, and intensity of the previous professional relationship.

REFERENCES

1. Council on Ethical and Judicial Affairs, American Medical Association. Sexual misconduct in the practice of medicine. JAMA. 1991;266:2741-5.
2. American College of Physicians. American College of Physicians Ethics Manual. Third edition. Ann Intern Med. 1992;117:947-60.
3. Gartrell N, Herman J, Olarte S, Feldstein M, Localio R. Psychiatrist-patient sexual contact: results of a national survey. I: Prevalence. Am J Psychiatry. 1986;143:1126-31.
4. Applebaum PS, Jorgenson L. Psychotherapist-patient sexual contact after termination of treatment: an analysis and a proposal. Am J Psychiatry. 1991;148:1466-73.

ANNOTATED BIBLIOGRAPHY

Council on Ethical and Judicial Affairs, American Medical Association. Sexual misconduct in the practice of medicine. JAMA. 1991;266:2741-5.

> Explains why the AMA says "just say no" to sex with patients and, in certain situations, with former patients. Encourages ethics education about physician–patient sex and rigorous reporting of sexual misconduct.

Johnson SH. Judicial review of disciplinary action for sexual misconduct in the practice of medicine. JAMA. 1993;270:1596-600.

> A lawyer looks at the legal implications of a professional ethic prohibiting sexual contact between physician and patient, plus early court cases.

White GE, Coverdale JA, Thomson AN. Can one be a good doctor and have a sexual relationship with one's patient? Fam Pract. 1994;11:389-93.

> Participants in a study of primary care physicians offer a range of definitions for sexual contact, social contact, and who constitutes a patient. Authors call for appropriate guidelines for physicians and better educational efforts through the teaching of medical students and through continuing medical education.

Part III

Medicine's Collective Obligations

No man is an island. No physician is an island in the sea of medicine. In addition to their primary duties to their individual patients, physicians have duties to patients collectively, to other physicians, and to society. Some of these duties are considered in this section. Two cases look at who physicians should or must accept as patients as an ethical matter (as apart from a legal one): Poor patients and HIV-infected and AIDS patients are discussed in Chapters 9 and 10, respectively. Chapter 11 examines the physician's duty to deal with an impaired colleague. The obligation to teach, and to teach well, the next generation of physicians and the responsibilities of medical residents are explored in Chapter 12, which looks at disagreements between residents and attendings, and in Chapter 13, which examines resident mistakes.

9

Ethics and Medicaid Patients

Commentary by LOIS SNYDER, JD
Case History by JANET WEINER, MPH,
and LOIS SNYDER, JD

CASE HISTORY

Harvey Mitchell, MD, is an internist in solo practice in a small city in the Northeast. One day he receives a message to call an old classmate, Linda Cohen, MD, who practices in an academic medical center at the other end of the state. The message indicates that Dr. Cohen would like to refer a patient named Bernadine Johnson, who is moving to Dr. Mitchell's area. Dr. Mitchell returns the call the next day, only to discover that Dr. Cohen is out of town. He tells Dr. Cohen's secretary that he would be happy to see Ms. Johnson and

Continued

to ask the patient to authorize the transfer of records. Dr. Mitchell tells his receptionist to schedule Ms. Johnson if she calls and also mentions it to his nurse, who often screens new patients over the phone to assess their needs.

A few days later, Dr. Mitchell's nurse buzzes his office. She says, "You remember that referral from Dr. Cohen you mentioned? Well, she just called for an appointment, and I said I'd get back to her. She has Medicaid, and it took me 20 minutes just to review all of her problems on the phone. In case you didn't know . . . she has poorly controlled diabetes with congestive heart failure; a chronic, non-healing foot ulcer; peripheral neuropathy; retinopathy; and recurrent urinary tract infections. She wants us to coordinate all her care and make appointments with the subspecialists she needs. What do you want me to do?" Dr. Mitchell sighs and says, "Tell her that we're not taking any new patients, and give her Dr. Perry's number."

The next day Dr. Cohen calls Dr. Mitchell. "Harvey, I just heard from Bernadine Johnson, who said she couldn't get an appointment at your office. Did your receptionist just make a mistake or what?" Dr. Mitchell hedges. "Well, it's been really busy here, and besides, it sounds like she would be better off with Dr. Perry, who works in the community health center."

"But Harvey, I referred her to you because her care is complex, and I trust your judgment as a physician. Do you only see a certain kind of patient? Why are you turning her away?" Dr. Cohen asks, her anger rising. "How can you justify discrimination?"

Dr. Mitchell remains calm. "This isn't about discrimination . . . it's that I just can't accept Medicaid patients. Look, don't judge me—I'm out here in private practice, and I lose money on every Medicaid patient, not to mention one with this many problems. Even if I see her, there's no way I can get her the consults she needs. Do you know how much Medicaid pays for an initial visit? You may not have to face economic realities in your situation, but I can't avoid them in mine."

Is Dr. Mitchell ethically justified in refusing to care for Ms. Johnson?

COMMENTARY

But in truth, one ought always to ask oneself what would happen if everyone did as one is doing . . .

JEAN-PAUL SARTRE

This commentary explores the ethical, not legal, obligations raised in this case and as such focuses on balancing professional duties with financial realities and the fulfillment of collective duties through individual actions.

The initiation of the patient–physician relationship is based on agreement about medical care for the patient. A physician may not discriminate against a class or category of patients who fall within his or her specialty; however, in the absence of an existing relationship, a physician is not ethically obligated to provide care to an individual except in specific situations, for example, in an emergency, under a contract, or when no other physician is available. So says the American College of Phycisians *Ethics Manual* (1). So what obligations apply here?

If Dr. Mitchell refused to care for all patients of a particular race, the case would clearly be one of unethical discrimination against a class. If he refused to care for a patient of that race because he knew from another physician, for example, of that patient's history of prescription drug fraud activities, the case would also be clear—no ethical obligation. But Dr. Mitchell says he cannot accept Ms. Johnson as a patient because she has Medicaid.

Clearly, Dr. Mitchell is not ethically obligated to accept all Medicaid patients into his practice. The context for deciding to accept any patient, that is, the current composition of a practice, is an important factor. Dr. Mitchell might already have many Medicaid patients or might be a regular volunteer at a free clinic. Also important is the selection process. Is it ethical for a physician to regularly use criteria other than clinical expertise and factors intrinsic to the patient–physician relationship in choosing patients? Would Dr. Mitchell be on the same moral footing when he refuses to accept new patients because their illness is not within his area of competence, because he does not speak their language, or because the patients do not have private insurance?

The American College of Physicians *Ethics Manual* states unequivocally that the welfare of the patient must take primacy over the physician's fiscal considerations (1); the manual is less clear, however, on the role of fiscal considerations in the physician's acceptance of a new patient.

In 1990, Medicaid reimbursement levels averaged 69% of Medicare prevailing charges (2) and an even smaller percentage of private insurance payments. A private practice could conceivably not be sustained on Medicaid reimbursement alone. Dr. Mitchell's decision is certainly ethical if accepting Medicaid threatens the viability of his practice (in which case, all of his patients will suffer). Ethics does not require that he accept all people who have Medicaid any more than he is required to work 18 hours a day to meet the needs of all potential patients. But does that mean he is ethically justified if he does not accept *any* Medicaid patients?

When Dr. Mitchell says "I lose money on every Medicaid patient," he probably means that Medicaid reimbursement does not cover his overhead costs, averaged out for each patient. General internists, however, see an average of 117 patients per week (3), and most of those patients do not have Medicaid. If Dr. Mitchell's practice is typical, the marginal cost of a few Medicaid patients would not threaten his practice or dramatically lower his overall income. The key lies in a fair and equitable distribution of Medicaid patients throughout medical practices. Physicians can satisfy both ethical and financial requirements by a commitment to this fair-share principle.

However, a 1992 report by the American Medical Association Council (AMA) on Ethical and Judicial Affairs stated that as many as one third of physicians provided little or no free or reduced-pay care and that "a disproportionate share of uncompensated care was provided by those practices which already had relatively high levels of Medicaid patients" (4). Some physicians are not seeing their fair share of the less profitable patient groups. If other physicians in the community are willing to accept Medicaid patients, are the physicians who do not accept them relieved of their obligation? How many physicians are referring patients to Dr. Perry at the community health center? Is it fair to colleagues for some physicians to avoid the less financially appealing patients, especially those needing complex care? Is it fair to the patients who get left out? Does this satisfy the collective obligation of the medical profession to society?

Some physicians might avoid this obligation in the belief that Medicaid patients are more likely to sue or for fear their presence in the waiting room will cause non-Medicaid patients to leave the practice (5, 6). But recent studies comparing medical malpractice claims made by Medicaid vs. non-Medicaid recipients do not support the belief that Medicaid patients are more litigious (6, 7). One physician whose practice includes many Medicaid patients had this to say about his patient mix: "Although many colleagues tell me 'off the record' that they shun Medicaid chiefly out of fear of losing private patients, I've found such defections to be largely a myth. Currently, about half my patients are Medicaid recipients, yet I've heard no complaints from the non-Medicaid segment" (5).

Although financial considerations are a fact of life, they should not interfere with the physician's primary commitment to patients. Reform that replaces our current patchwork approach to health care with a cohesive and coherent system that provides adequate access to care for all Americans is much needed. Reimbursement is most properly dealt with as a policy matter at the system level—not at the level of physician and patient.

As a practical matter, any given patient probably ultimately receives care, albeit perhaps after being shuffled from physician to physician or to a clinic. Or the patient might end up in an emergency room. The consequent delay in care can hurt patients and is inefficient. To enter the medical profession is to recognize the obligation to participate in medicine's collective responsibility to all who are sick and to ensure that resources are used wisely. Otherwise, the profession has a collective duty that no single physician is obligated to fulfill. Where once the profession taught its students and young physicians the "ancient message that a physician is bound by 'professing' humane kindness (humanitas) and compassion (misericordia) to those in need," one physician has noted that any sense of obligation to care for the poor is diminishing and that, as a consequence, the cynicism of both physicians and patients is fueled when young physicians are taught that they may put their own financial interests ahead of patient needs (8).

This cynicism is fueled further by the reluctance on the part of some physicians to be honest about their reasons for refusing patients. As in this case study, if a "wrong" answer is given to an appointment secretary's inquiry about insurance or ability to pay, then there can suddenly be no room in the doctor's schedule for a new patient. This phenomenon has been examined as it applies to Medicare patients (9). Obviously, lying to a prospective patient or the referring physician about the reason for not accepting the individual cannot be condoned. Truth telling is a basic tenet of the medical profession and is essential to relationships with colleagues and patients and to the social contract within which medicine is practiced.

Every physician should participate in implementing the fair-share principle. Accomplishing this task can be done by providing care to the poor in the office setting at no or reduced cost, serving at clinics that treat the poor or at shelters for homeless persons or abused women, accepting Medicaid patients in sufficient numbers, or participating in programs developed by medical societies to care for those in need.

How much is fair? The AMA Council on Ethical and Judicial Affairs has said the following:

"The measure of what constitutes an appropriate contribution may vary with circumstances such as community characteristics, geographic location, the nature of the physician's practice and specialty, and other conditions. All physicians should work to ensure that the needs of the poor in their communities are met. Caring for the poor should become a normal part of the physician's overall service to patients.

"In the poorest communities, it may not be possible to meet the needs of the indigent for physicians' services by relying solely on local physicians. The local physicians should be able to turn for assistance to their colleagues in prosperous communities, particularly those in close proximity.

"State, local, and specialty medical societies should help physicians meet their obligations to provide care to the indigent" (4).

Dr. Mitchell might have decided long ago that he would not accept any Medicaid patients. Or he might have a waiting room with many Medicaid patients and merely be refusing to accept another. We do not know. We do know, however, that based on a fair-share principle, the latter explanation seems ethically defensible while the former does not.

REFERENCES

1. American College of Physicians. American College of Physicians Ethics Manual. Third edition. Ann Intern Med. 1992;117:947-60.
2. Physician Payment Review Commission. Annual Report to Congress 1991. Washington, D.C.: Physician Payment Review Commission; 1991.
3. American Medical Association. Physician Marketplace Statistics 1991. Chicago: American Medical Association; 1991.
4. American Medical Association. Caring for the poor. JAMA. 1993; 269:2533-7.
5. Attwood C. It's unfair—and unwise—to shun Medicaid patients. Medical Economics. 1991;68:22,24-5,28.
6. McNulty M. Questions and answers: are poor patients likely to sue for malpractice? JAMA. 1989;262:1391-2.
7. Mussman MG, Zawistowich L, Weisman CS, Malitz FE, Morlock LL. Medical malpractice claims filed by Medicaid and non-Medicaid recipients in Maryland. JAMA. 1991;265:2992-4.
8. Miles SH. What are we teaching about indigent patients? JAMA. 1992;268:2562-3.
9. Butler RN. Doctors are refusing to treat Medicare patients. The Washington Post. 1992; May 12.

ANNOTATED BIBLIOGRAPHY

American Medical Association. Caring for the poor. JAMA. 1993;269: 2533-7.

The AMA takes a historical look at how the poor have been cared for, identifies current problems, and finds that every physician has a duty to share in providing care to indigent persons and that medical societies should assist physicians in meeting this responsibility.

Gordon HL, Reiser SJ. Do physicians have a duty to treat Medicare patients? Arch Intern Med. 1993;153:563-5.

Examines arguments for and against accepting Medicare patients, asserts that all doctors should serve the patient, including Medicare patients, but also calls for changes in Medicare to ease economic and administrative barriers to care.

Miles SH. What are we teaching about indigent patients? JAMA. 1992;268:2562-3.

Uses a case study to explore physician obligations and the message being sent to physicians in training when hospitals transfer patients on the basis of their inability to pay. Finds that fiscal limits on patient care go beyond simple practice environment issues to pose basic ethical questions and choices for medicine as a profession. An eloquent call to arms.

10

The Duty to Treat
HIV-Positive Patients

Case History and Commentary by JANET WEINER, MPH

CASE HISTORY

John Alden, age 40, has chronic, stable angina that does not respond to medical therapies. He makes a return visit to Dr. Standish, an internist who has followed Mr. Alden for five years. Dr. Standish finds, while taking the patient's interval history, that Mr. Alden was tested for HIV a year ago at an anonymous site and is HIV-positive. Mr. Alden reports that he feels well, in general, but has noticed significant worsening of his chest pain. His physical examination is unchanged. Because of the change in Mr. Alden's cardiac symptoms, Dr. Standish orders an exercise thallium scan, which suggests two-vessel involvement.

Continued

71

Dr. Standish refers Mr. Alden to Dr. Montgomery, head of cardiology at Sheridan Hospital, for a same-day catheterization. Dr. Montgomery, in reviewing the medical records, notes that Mr. Alden is HIV-positive. He tells Dr. Standish that he and his staff have decided to refuse to do elective cardiac catheterizations on HIV-positive patients. Dr. Standish is shocked and accuses Dr. Montgomery of gross dereliction of his duty to patients.

Dr. Montgomery is offended. He claims that the risk of HIV transmission to his staff far outweighs the benefits of the procedure to the patient, especially in the long term. He explains that this decision was not made lightly but was in response to the recent discovery that his chief resident contracted HIV after exposure to the virus during a procedure. Subsequently, the entire medical staff petitioned the hospital to test all patients for HIV on admission. The request was denied because of legal concerns and inadequate counseling services for HIV-positive patients.

The medical staff strongly believes that universal precautions do not adequately protect physicians doing invasive procedures. Also, the house staff has no life or disability insurance in the event of HIV infection. Because the hospital is in an area of high HIV prevalence, the staff deemed these risks unacceptably high. Dr. Montgomery says that the hospital administration, while not fully agreeing with this position, supports the staff's decision. He believes Mr. Alden's best interests would be served by referring him to another cardiac care center.

On hearing all of this, Dr. Standish is somewhat sympathetic but fails to be persuaded. He cannot follow Mr. Alden through catheterization, possible surgery, and recovery at another hospital where he has no privileges. He wonders what to say to Mr. Alden and what this experience tells him about voluntary HIV testing.

COMMENTARY

The College, among other groups, has upheld the physician's duty to treat AIDS and HIV-positive patients, drawing on the professionalism of medicine. "It is inappropriate for any health care professional to compromise the treatment of any patient, including those with transmissible, lethal diseases such as AIDS, on the grounds that such patients present unacceptable medical risks" (1). The American College of Physicians *Ethics Manual* states that "a physician may not discriminate against a class or category of patients . . . " (2).

This case study illustrates the difficulties and conflicts physicians may face in fulfilling their obligations to patients. In practical terms, no obligation is absolute. What are the boundaries of this duty to treat, and how can ethical parameters guide individual physicians in the wake of AIDS?

The ethical imperative to treat AIDS patients stems from the duty to treat all classes of patients within a physician's sphere of competence. Although a physician is not obligated to treat any one patient (except in certain circumstances such as in an emergency room or on call), refusing to treat entire groups of people violates the values of professional responsibility.

Contrast this principle with a more commercial model of physician responsibility, in which physicians are not obligated to treat any person or group. In this model, medicine is more like a trade; physicians are business people who sell their skills to consumers (patients) and become obligated only through contractual arrangements (3).

The College has consistently rejected the commercial model as the sole interpretation of the physician–patient relationship. "The practice of medicine is a societal trust and carries with it a societal responsibility. If medicine wishes to retain its respected status as the healing profession, we must continue to provide the best possible care to our patients, regardless of risk" (1).

Assuming that the physicians in this example accept this notion of professional responsibility, how can we understand their different positions? Dr. Standish wants to provide the best care he can to Mr. Alden by referring him appropriately and following him through the length of his hospital stay and recovery. He believes that Mr. Alden's HIV status does not preclude an elective workup of angina because the patient is asymptomatic (for HIV infection) and is likely to live many years. As a general internist, Dr. Standish does not do invasive procedures and believes universal precautions adequately protect him from HIV infection.

Dr. Montgomery, on the other hand, runs the cardiac catheterization lab, where parenteral blood exposures occur frequently. One staff member has already seroconverted, and Dr. Montgomery has heard estimates of a 0.5% to 12% annual risk for infection for surgeons and other physicians doing invasive procedures in high prevalence areas (4, 5). He believes the cumulative mortality risk is unacceptable for his staff, especially when weighed against the marginal benefits of certain invasive procedures to many HIV-positive patients.

However, recent data do not support the magnitude of risk that Dr. Montgomery presupposes. The cumulative risk for HIV infection in health care workers depends on three variables: the prevalence of the virus in the patient population; the frequency of needlestick exposures; and the risk for seroconversion from a single contaminated needlestick (5).

In a study of surgical personnel at San Francisco General Hospital, Gerberding and colleagues calculated a theoretical risk for occupational HIV infection of 0.125 infections per year, or one infection among surgical personnel every eight years (6). As the authors state, even this level of risk represents a major life-threatening occupational hazard for surgical personnel at San Francisco General. In places of average (less than 3%) HIV prevalence, the risk would be reduced to one infection among the surgical staff every 80 years.

Dr. Montgomery also confuses the equation in medical decision making by weighing the risks to the physician against the benefits to the patient. Clinical indications consist of the patient's risks and benefits; although an elective cardiac workup may not be indicated for an acutely ill AIDS patient, that decision is based on medical futility (itself a complex, controversial issue). Dr. Montgomery would have to prove that the prognosis for Mr. Alden makes the workup futile— an untenable position these days.

Nevertheless, Dr. Montgomery does have a moral responsibility to minimize the risk to his staff. He is on more solid ethical footing if the results of routine HIV testing are used to manage risk without compromising patient care. These circumstances are realized only if evidence indicates that physician knowledge of patients' HIV status reduces risk to the medical staff and if all patients give truly informed consent. There is some evidence against the first point; in fact, some commentators have suggested that HIV testing of patients will put physicians at greater risk because they will be reassured by negative results, some of which will be false.

Lastly, Dr. Montgomery believes that the current climate of fear and hesitation at Sheridan Hospital, given the chief resident's seroconversion, precludes providing optimal care to Mr. Alden. Since there are several other cardiac care centers nearby, he does not feel that he has abrogated his professional responsibility to patients, but he does feel he has achieved a delicate balance between his "duty to treat" and his moral obligation to his staff.

Dr. Standish cannot agree. While he acknowledges that Mr. Alden can get good care at another hospital, he does not believe that the staff at Sheridan Hospital has fulfilled its duties. He recognizes that referring his patient elsewhere may be the best compromise in this instance. But his patient may suffer from the discontinuity of care and spend more time and money traveling to another center. Dr. Standish is also concerned about the staff's categorical refusal to treat HIV-positive patients. How can medicine as a profession meet its collective obligation to patients if all physicians do not share the burden?

The "duty to treat" has little meaning if fear or inexperience excuses physicians from their responsibilities. It is disingenuous, and somewhat circular, for a physician to claim that fear of a class of patients precludes optimal and justifies refusing to treat the entire class. Fear and deliberate inexperience can interfere with patient care, but physicians have a moral responsibility to confront and overcome personal barriers and not just to refer patients to other physicians.

In turn, medical institutions have a responsibility to minimize the actual and perceived risk to their medical staffs. As one HIV-positive resident wrote, "A safe work environment also means one in which health workers are well protected economically, with appropriate health, disability, and life insurance" (7). Sheridan Hospital might arrange lectures and discussions about HIV and its transmission; train the staff in universal precautions and stress strict adherence to them; invite the staff to suggest further precautions that might enhance safety without compromising patient care; and review life and disability coverage to ensure adequate financial protection for the entire staff.

Finally, after confronting fear and overcoming inexperience, physicians must grapple with the bounds of acceptable risk. Some risks are too great even for dedicated professionals. Soldiers are not duty-bound to perform suicide missions nor are firefighters required to enter buildings that are on the verge of collapse (5). The occupational risk of HIV transmission should be judged relative to risks faced by other professionals and to other risks faced by physicians.

Conflicts surrounding hazardous duty have existed as long as the medical profession itself. History reveals that physicians struggled with ethical conduct in the face of epidemics such as bubonic plague, yellow fever, smallpox, and cholera and were often surrounded by large and largely unexplored risks to their lives (8). Some physicians fled or refused to treat the victims; others cared selflessly for all the sick, and some died with their patients.

So while occupational risk is not new to physicians, AIDS has introduced the problem to generations of health professionals relatively unaccustomed to confronting real personal danger as they deliver medical care. The stigma of the diagnosis, the devastation of the illness itself, and persistent media attention have combined to highlight this occupational risk above all others.

In fact, physicians are at far greater risk for hepatitis B and tuberculosis infection than for HIV infection. An estimated 12,000 health care workers become infected yearly with the hepatitis B virus, and 250 of these eventually die from it (9). Of all health care workers, 15% to 30% show evidence of exposure to hepatitis B, which is far more infectious than HIV. The risk for HIV infection after needlestick exposure to contaminated blood is 0.5% compared with 6% to 30% for hepatitis B. Despite the availability of a fairly effective vaccine, many physicians do not protect themselves against hepatitis B infection (10). Clearly, physicians accept this level of occupational risk, and refusing to treat HIV-positive patients must be viewed in this context. The rising incidence of AIDS has provoked a degree of fear unparalleled in recent memory, a fear to which physicians are not immune.

In a recent national survey (11), 75% of 2450 physician respondents agreed with the following statement: "A physician may not ethically refuse to treat a patient whose condition is within the physician's current realm of competence solely because the patient is seropositive (for HIV)." However, there were statistically significant differences among and within specialties. General internists (85%) were more likely than internal medicine subspecialists (73%) to agree with the statement. Although the precise reasons for this pattern are unclear, the authors noted that many medical subspecialists perform procedures that may increase their perceived risk. General surgeons (69%), surgical specialists (59%), and obstetrician-gynecologists (64%) were less likely to feel that physicians have an ethical responsibility to treat HIV-positive patients.

The increase in AIDS cases offers us a critical test of the ethical parameters of the duty to treat as well as an opportunity to reaffirm medical values and principles. In accord with societal and professional standards, the College reaffirms the ethical imperative to deliver quality care to HIV-positive and AIDS patients.

REFERENCES

1. American College of Physicians and the Infectious Disease Society of America. The acquired immunodeficiency syndrome (AIDS) and infection with the human immunodeficiency virus (HIV). Ann Intern Med. 1988;108:460-9.
2. American College of Physicians. American College of Physicians Ethics Manual, Part 1. Ann Intern Med. 1989;111:245-52.
3. Annas GJ. Not saints, but healers: the legal duties of health care professionals in the AIDS epidemic. Am J Public Health. 1988;78:844-9.
4. Task Force on AIDS and Orthopedic Surgery. Recommendations for the Prevention of Human Immunodeficiency Virus (HIV) Transmission in the Practice of Orthopedic Surgery. American Academy of Orthopedic Surgeons, July 1989.
5. Emanuel EJ. Do physicians have an obligation to treat patients with AIDS? N Engl J Med. 1988;318:1686-90.
6. Gerberding JL, Littell C, Tarkington A, Brown A, Schecter WP. Risk of exposure of surgical personnel to patients' blood during surgery at San Francisco General Hospital. N Engl J Med. 1990;322:1788-93.
7. Aoun H. When a house officer gets AIDS. N Engl J Med. 1989;321:693-6.
8. Zuger A, Miles SH. AIDS and occupational risk. Historic traditions and ethical obligations. JAMA. 1987;258:1924-8.
9. Centers for Disease Control. Guidelines for the prevention of transmis-

sion of human immunodeficiency virus and hepatitis B virus to health-care and public-safety workers. MMWR Morb Mortal Wkly Rep. 1989;38:S-6.
10. ACP Task Force on Adult Immunization and Infectious Diseases Society of America. Guide for Adult Immunization. Third edition. Philadelphia: American College of Physicians; 1994.
11. Rizzo JA, Marder WD, Willke RJ. Physician contact with and attitudes toward HIV-seropositive patients. Results from a national survey. Med Care. 1990;28:251-60.

ANNOTATED BIBLIOGRAPHY

Annas GJ. Not saints, but healers: the legal duties of health care profession-als in the AIDS epidemic. Am J Public Health. 1988;78:844-9.

> Reviews legal history and thought; provides a framework for encour-aging the duty to treat as a matter of ethics.

Cooke M. Patient rights and physician responsibility: four problems in AIDS care. In: Volberding P, Jacobson MA, eds. AIDS Clinical Review 1993/1994. New York: Marcel Dekker, Inc.; 1994.

> Encourages expansion of the number of providers willing to treat HIV-infected patients under a section on the right to receive care. Also includes sections on the right to control the medical record, the right to experimental therapies, and the right to die.

Emanuel EJ. Do physicians have an obligation to treat patients with AIDS? N Engl J Med. 1988;318:1686-90.

> The author says "yes." Although this responsibility can be tempered by factors such as excessive risk, the author argues that individual physicians have this obligation as members of a learned profession who care for the ill.

Gerbert BG, Maguire BT, Bleecker T, Coates TJ, McPhee SJ. Primary care physicians and AIDS: attitudinal and structural barriers to care. JAMA. 1991;266:2837-42.

> Survey of primary care physicians found that most believed in a duty to treat HIV-infected patients, but it also found obstacles to care such as negativity toward certain patient groups and time constraints that limit care.

Zuger A, Miles SH. Physicians, AIDS and occupational risk. Historic tradi-tions and ethical obligations. JAMA. 1987;258:1924-8.

> Examines physician responses to other deadly contagious diseases and affirms a duty to treat patients with AIDS because medicine is a moral enterprise.

11

The Impaired Colleague

Commentary by JANET WEINER, MPH, and LOIS SNYDER, JD
Case History by JANET WEINER, MPH

CASE HISTORY

Paul Daniels, MD, is an associate professor of medicine at General Hospital. He is well known for his clinical and diagnostic skills and has many patients referred to him because their cases are clinical "puzzles." He has been at General Hospital for 10 years, through internship and residency, and is respected within the institution.

Carla Martin, MD, is a recently appointed assistant professor of medicine at General Hospital. At a Saturday faculty party, Dr. Martin notices that Dr. Daniels is slurring his words and staggering; she is concerned about Dr. Daniels driving home while

Continued

intoxicated. He assures her that he is sober and can drive safely.

During this conversation, Dr. Daniels' beeper goes off, and he answers his page. Dr. Martin overhears the discussion between Dr. Daniels and a new intern and realizes that Dr. Daniels is on call. She hears Dr. Daniels prescribe an unusually large dose of digoxin for the patient in question. When Dr. Martin asks Dr. Daniels about the patient, he says the problem is routine and that the new intern has July-itis.

Dr. Martin worries all weekend about the patient on digoxin. On Monday morning, she finds the patient and reviews the chart. The intern did not follow Dr. Daniels' instructions and gave the patient a much lower dose. Dr. Martin tracks down the intern and asks about the digoxin dosage. The young intern says that she checked with a more senior resident because she thought she misheard Dr. Daniels' directions and had given the lower dosage on the resident's instructions. Dr. Martin assures the apologetic intern that she gave the patient the correct dosage but does not tell her about Dr. Daniels' mistake.

That day, Dr. Martin tries to discuss the issue with Dr. Daniels, who tells her that she is completely out of line. He denies any inappropriate behavior or having a drinking problem. He questions Dr. Martin's motives and tells her to mind her own business.

Dr. Martin makes discreet inquiries about Dr. Daniels and discovers that other faculty members have noticed him drinking excessively at parties. In fact, his friends on the staff often draw straws to decide who will drive him home after a party. No one seems concerned about Dr. Daniels' clinical competence. As Dr. Martin decides what to do, she looks into programs at General Hospital for employees with substance abuse problems. She finds that General Hospital has had a voluntary, confidential program in place for 10 years. When a physician is involved, an immediate assessment is made of the physician's clinical competence and threat to patient safety. Clinical performance is monitored directly.

Dr. Martin is unsure about her next steps. Being relatively new to General Hospital, she questions her interpretation of Dr. Daniels' behavior. Other faculty members, who have known Dr. Daniels for a long time, seem unconcerned about his drinking. What should she do?

———◆———

COMMENTARY

This case study highlights the difficult issues surrounding the professional mandate to protect patients from physicians impaired by psychiatric, physiologic, or physical disorders. The American College of Physicians *Ethics Manual* is firm: "It is the responsibility of every physician to protect the public from an impaired physician. . . . All steps must be taken to assure that no patient is harmed because of actions or decisions made by an impaired physician" (1). But upholding this duty often necessitates making a judgment about a colleague's impairment as well as confronting institutional, social, and personal barriers.

In this case study, Dr. Martin has direct evidence that a patient could have been harmed by Dr. Daniels' actions. She might not be in the best position to judge the level of his impairment since she has limited experience with Dr. Daniels and is new to the institution. Nevertheless, it is her moral duty to ensure that his impairment and clinical competence are assessed by an appropriate authority.

Dr. Daniels should be confronted again and told to seek help, particularly through General Hospital's voluntary, confidential program. Dr. Martin could try this type of confrontation again, or she could inform the appropriate parties within the institution (possibly the division or department chief) about the incident she witnessed and her conversation with the young intern. If the institutional authorities fail to act, Dr. Martin should consider reporting Dr. Daniels to the state medical society. Most societies have impaired physician programs.

We can envision the dilemmas facing Dr. Martin as she tries to fulfill her obligations. In General Hospital, Dr. Daniels is respected, well-known, and tenured; Dr. Martin is a relatively new faculty member whose future at the hospital could be at stake. She might also have a normal aversion to confrontation, especially about a topic as sensitive as physician impairment. She might worry about losing the respect and trust of her peers and about the legal implications of making such an accusation. Clearly, Dr. Martin takes a certain risk, personally and professionally, by pursuing this issue.

But confronting Dr. Daniels, or reporting him, need not be seen exclusively in a negative light. Great progress has been made in treating impaired physicians in recent years, ever since the American Medical Association (AMA) produced its landmark report "The Sick Physician." In 1973, the AMA adopted the program recommended in its report, which stressed the physician's ethical obligation to help impaired colleagues while ensuring that impaired physicians do not endanger patients (2). Most programs now emphasize treatment and rehabilitation rather than discipline and sanctions. And recovery rates for physicians are higher than those in the general population: In a case-control study, 83% of physicians had returned to practice and were functioning well 3 years after treatment compared with 62% of non-physician, middle-class control subjects (2).

Dr. Martin may also worry about her legal duties and protection. While statutes vary from state to state, many states have instituted "snitch laws" that require certain groups of people (such as physician colleagues and health care entities) to report knowledge of physician impairment to either a state medical society or licensing board (3).

Most laws provide a certain degree of anonymity for reporting parties as well as immunity from a civil suit but at the same time set penalties for those designated who do not report an impaired physician. Most laws also allow for confidentiality of the impaired physician's records. Dr. Martin should contact her state medical society to find out the legal requirements in her state.

Regardless of Dr. Martin's legal duties, she is morally required to protect patients from harm. She must resist a natural impulse to remain uninvolved—especially given that Dr. Daniels is senior to her—or to identify with him. Certainly, she should act carefully and discreetly, but she must also take definitive action.

How far does Dr. Martin's obligation extend? If Dr. Daniels agrees to seek treatment, how can Dr. Martin be sure he goes? Is it appropriate for her to check? If she reports Dr. Daniels to the department head, is her obligation fulfilled even if that person fails to act? In other words, when has Dr. Martin done enough?

We do not see easy answers to these questions. There may be practical limits to what Dr. Martin can do within her institution and in her role as Dr. Daniels' colleague. One person cannot be completely responsible for the actions of another. However, the following rule is a reasonable guide: A physician's obligation corresponds to how much evidence exists that a patient could be harmed.

In our case study, Dr. Martin knows that a patient could have been harmed, and she should assume that Dr. Daniels' other patients are at risk. Thus, her obligation extends further than if she had only noticed Dr. Daniels drinking excessively at a party when he was not on call. In that case, expressing her concern to Dr. Daniels only and remaining alert to other signs of Dr. Daniels' potential impairment might have been sufficient.

Although we have emphasized Dr. Martin's ethical obligations here, we do not minimize Dr. Daniels' responsibility for his own behavior. He clearly violated the maxim *primum non nocere*—"first, do no harm"—which has been a cornerstone of physician ethics for centuries.

Beyond the direct threat to patient safety, Dr. Daniels' drinking could also have dire consequences for the young interns and residents he supervises.

Clearly, Dr. Daniels bears the ultimate responsibility for his impairment. But this acknowledgment should not obscure the nature of Dr. Daniels' problem, which is substance abuse. At every step, the ultimate goal of all parties—the impaired physician, knowing colleagues, and institutional programs—is protection of patients, followed by rehabilitation of the impaired physician and a return to clinical competence.

REFERENCES

1. American College of Physicians. American College of Physicians Ethics Manual. Third edition. Ann Intern Med. 1992;117:947-60.
2. Sargent DA. The impaired physician movement: an interim report. Hosp Community Psychiatry. 1985;36:294-7.
3. Walzer RS. Impaired physicians: an overview and update of the legal issues. J Leg Med. 1990;11:131-98.

ANNOTATED BIBLIOGRAPHY

Centrella M. Physician addiction and impairment—current thinking: a review. J Addict Dis. 1994;13:91-105.

> Looks at definitions, prevalence, diagnosis, treatment, rehabilitation, prevention, and other aspects of physician impairment with an emphasis on what works.

Deckard G, Meterko M, Field D. Physician burnout: an examination of personal, professional, and organizational relationships. Med Care. July 1994;32:745-54.

> Empirically assesses burnout among staff model HMO doctors and recommends that organizations review policies, procedures, and management structures that contribute to high rates of emotional exhaustion and other manifestations of burnout.

Morreim H. Am I my brother's warden? Responding to the unethical or incompetent colleague. Hastings Cent Rep. 1993;23:19-27.

> Argues that physicians must care for their own and respond to unethical or incompetent colleagues lest the integrity of the entire profession be compromised. Points out the incentives to not get involved, but exhorts that physicians must take responsibility for self-regulation.

12

When Residents and Attendings Disagree

Case History and Commentary by ERROL D. CROOK, MD, and JANET WEINER, MPH

CASE HISTORY

Two months ago, Mr. Jones, who is age 60 and a cigarette smoker, was diagnosed with unresectable squamous cell carcinoma of the lung. He had previously been in good health and had not seen a doctor in years. Unfortunately, the plant he had worked in for several years recently closed, and he could not afford to continue his medical insurance.

Susan Shaw, MD, an internal medicine resident rotating on the oncology service for two months, took care of Mr. Jones at the county hospital when the diagnosis was made and has since seen him twice in the oncology clinic. At these visits, Mr. Jones rarely saw an

Continued

attending physician and considered Dr. Shaw to be his doctor. After extensive discussion with Dr. Shaw about the diagnosis, Mr. Jones and his wife decided on palliative therapy as the only form of treatment, although no written advance directive was created. Because Dr. Shaw plans to become an oncologist, the attendings knew her well and agreed with her plans for Mr. Jones.

Until one week ago, Mr. Jones had been doing relatively well and had been quite active. Since then, however, he has experienced progressive shortness of breath, malaise, and a productive cough. After developing fever and chills, he comes to the emergency department seeking relief from his symptoms. Dr. Shaw is on call and is paged to the emergency department to evaluate Mr. Jones. She diagnoses post-obstructive pneumonia and orders antibiotics and oxygen, which moderately relieve Mr. Jones' severe shortness of breath and hypoxemia. A few hours later she returns to check on him. He still has to work hard to breathe, despite the high concentration of oxygen being delivered. Recognizing that Mr. Jones' condition could very possibly worsen over the next several hours, Dr. Shaw sits down to discuss Mr. Jones' wishes with him.

Dr. Shaw informs Mr. Jones that his illness is severe and could lead to the need for mechanical ventilation. She tells him that some forms of therapy might relieve his obstruction and improve his chances of recovery. Despite his severe illness, Mr. Jones listens attentively and understands his options. He decides that he would rather not be intubated for any reason. He also decides against any form of therapy other than antibiotics to treat his pneumonia and oxygen to relieve his dyspnea. He says that he has had a good life and has come to terms with his illness.

Dr. Shaw makes note of Mr. Jones' decision; she feels comfortable with his decision, knowing that he came to it after careful analysis of all of the information given to him. He has shown clear reasoning. She feels confident that his decision is based on a desire to live out his life without aggressive medical care and not on external or financial considerations.

The next morning Dr. Shaw introduces Mr. Jones to her attending, Barry Davis, MD. She tells Dr. Davis of Mr. Jones' wishes not to be intubated and to forgo therapy other than antibiotics and oxygen. After reviewing the case and the x-rays, Dr. Davis feels that localized external beam radiation would relieve Mr. Jones' obstruction and that he would probably recover from his pneumonia. Mr. Jones had been doing well—given his diagnosis—before this acute illness, which is in his favor. Dr. Davis decides to convince Mr. Jones to try the more aggressive approach.

The two doctors have a lengthy conversation with Mr. Jones about his tumor and pneumonia. Mr. Jones, who is in even more respiratory distress than before, stands by his earlier decision. Dr. Davis does not feel comfortable with the decision and asks Dr. Shaw to call the pulmonologist and radiation oncologist to see Mr. Jones. She asks why. Dr. Davis says he feels that Mr. Jones is giving up and may be denying himself several weeks to months of life. He does not think the patient can make a rational decision given the severity of his acute illness, and in cases like this, he would rather be aggressive. "I've seen patients change their minds as they became increasingly ill, but by then it may be too late," Dr. Davis says.

Dr. Shaw disagrees with Dr. Davis' approach. She thinks that calling in consultants is a breach of Mr. Jones' well-thought-out wishes. How should Dr. Shaw handle her disagreement with Dr. Davis' plan?

———⟫◆⟪———

COMMENTARY

This case raises several important issues, including the ethical responsibilities of physicians-in-training regarding patient advocacy and end-of-life decision making. First, let's explore Dr. Shaw's position as an internal medicine resident who disagrees with the attending physician's plan. Dr. Shaw is the physician with the longest and closest relationship with the patient, who depends on her for guidance in making medical decisions. Mr. Jones considers Dr. Shaw his doctor and his biggest supporter in the medical system. The role of patient advocate, foreign to many residents, carries serious obligations.

Dr. Shaw's dual role as physician-in-training and patient advocate has caused personal conflict. As a resident, she does not have the power to make final decisions about a patient's care. And to argue vigorously for Mr. Jones' wishes could cause problems for her since she will be applying for oncology fellowships in the near future. What are her options and obligations?

The Amerian College of Physicians *Ethics Manual* states that "Residents . . . are bound by the same ethical principles as other physicians [and] should acknowledge their limitations and ask for help or supervision from the attending physician, chief of service, or consultants when concerns arise about patient care . . . " (1). What is best for the patient must be the primary concern, and the patient's wishes must be respected. Therefore, Dr. Shaw should continue discussions with the patient and her attending.

She must be sure that Mr. Jones' decision is, in fact, what he really wants. He has to understand the risks and benefits of any possible therapy as well as the consequences of refusing therapy. To this end, the consultations requested by Dr. Davis may be beneficial— not in a persuasive manner as Dr. Davis would like but in an educational sense. The consultants will provide Mr. Jones with the most complete data available about his prognosis and options, including details Dr. Shaw may not have had. Dr. Shaw, as patient advocate, must be sure that any decision Mr. Jones makes is truly informed.

Dr. Shaw should also discuss her concerns directly with Dr. Davis. His experience gives him a unique perspective that Dr. Shaw might find eye opening. As an oncologist, he deals with end-of-life decisions frequently. His actions are likely based on experience in this kind of situation, which he has faced far more often than Dr. Shaw has. Dr. Davis knows that if Mr. Jones eventually changes his mind, his chances of surviving this episode might be slimmer because of the delay in starting therapy. The *Ethics Manual* supports a physician's right to persuade, if he or she feels it is unwise for a patient to refuse therapy, but not to coerce. The manual states, "Physicians have the obligation to ensure that the refusal is truly informed, to give a clear recommendation, and to try to persuade the patient, but ultimately they must accept the patient's decision" (1).

A discussion between both physicians, in addition to being educational, would give Dr. Shaw an opportunity to relay Mr. Jones' and her concerns to Dr. Davis. In turn, Dr. Davis should respect the relationship between Dr. Shaw and Mr. Jones and give credence to Dr. Shaw's insights. Although she has not had a long-standing relationship with the patient, the length of the relationship is not as critical as the content of their interactions.

To carry the scenario a step further: After consultations and discussions, Dr. Davis continues to try to persuade Mr. Jones to change his mind. Dr. Shaw finds herself in an even more complicated position. Because she is the only physician with an established relationship with Mr. Jones, she must continue to act on his behalf. Using the guidelines stated above, she should seek help from her chief resident or program director. She could also consult the chief of staff or the hospital ethics committee or broach the issue at noon conference or morning report. Dr. Shaw's options would vary from institution to institution, and she should use tact and diplomacy in deciding who to involve first. What is best for the patient must remain primary, although Dr. Shaw is vulnerable as a resident and future oncology fellow.

Should Dr. Shaw withdraw from the case? The *Ethics Manual* allows for residents to withdraw from cases in which there may be ethical or religious concerns, after in-depth discussion with the attending physician and arrangement of alternative coverage (1). However, for Dr. Shaw to withdraw from this case would not be appropriate, given her relationship with the patient and his family. Withdrawal may be warranted in cases in which the resident has moral objections to therapy that the patient or family wants. For example, a resident may be opposed to withdrawing tube feeding, even if the patient and family insist on it and others agree. In our case, Dr. Shaw has no moral conflict with the patient's wishes and should continue in her role as patient advocate.

This case also points out the potential benefits of completing an advance directive in the outpatient setting. The Patient Self-Determination Act of 1990 requires most health care institutions to inform patients on admission about their right to complete an advance directive. However, this requirement is no substitute for discussions and written directives at outpatient visits before the patient is acutely ill. With ". . . advance directives, competent patients state what treatments they would accept or decline if they lost decision-making capacity . . . patients also indicate their general goals for care" (1). Mr. Jones came to the hospital without a formal advance directive, although he had limited discussions with Dr. Shaw in the clinic.

Why did Mr. Jones not complete a written advance directive before he was hospitalized? He faced several possible barriers: He did not have a primary care physician with whom he had had a long relationship. His "doctor"—Dr. Shaw—met him during one hospitalization, saw him only twice in the clinic, and is on this clinical service rotation for only a short time. These same barriers contributed to the conflicts during his hospitalization. The attending physician of record has not had extensive conversations with the patient, yet bears the ultimate responsibility for the treatment plan.

A written advance directive would become operative only if Mr. Jones were no longer competent. It would not prevent a mentally competent Mr. Jones from changing his mind during hospitalization as treatment options were presented to him. And it does not mean that he wants to refuse all treatment and medical care. In each situation, the physician needs to discuss with the patient (or a surrogate, if the patient is incompetent) any treatment, whether palliative, curative, or resuscitative in nature.

In sum, Dr. Shaw should explore several options to resolve her problem. She must be sure that Mr. Jones is well informed and consistent in his decision. She may need further guidance from a chief resident or program officer but should express her concerns directly to Dr. Davis. Her primary obligation is to the patient, who considers her his strongest advocate. If Mr. Jones continues to decline further treatment, his comfort should be assured and his wishes respected.

REFERENCE

1. American College of Physicians. American College of Physicians Ethics Manual. Third edition. Ann Intern Med. 1992;117:947-60.

ANNOTATED BIBLIOGRAPHY

Christakis DA, Feudtner C. Ethics in a short white coat: the ethical dilemmas that medical students confront. Acad Med. 1993;68:249-54; and Making the rounds: the ethical development of medical students in the context of clinical rotations. Hastings Cent Rep. 1994;24:6-12.

These articles examine clinical ethics dilemmas that medical students face and call for educational efforts geared specifically to medical students as well as to residents and attendings.

13

Medical Residents, Attendings, and Mistakes

Commentary by ANNE-MARIE AUDET, MD, and JANET
WEINER, MPH
Case History by ANNE-MARIE AUDET, MD

CASE HISTORY

It is late Friday night at Mercy Hospital. Martha
Ellsworth, MD, the intern on call for the general medicine service, is paged to the emergency room. There
she sees Mr. Friend, a 68-year-old man who needs to
be admitted for treatment of acute bronchospasm.

Mr. Friend has a history of hypertension, adult-
onset diabetes mellitus, and asthma. For the past
week, he has been visiting his daughter, who has a
dog, and he noticed he was having increased difficulty breathing. Tonight, he could not sleep and became

Continued

progressively distressed because he could not "get any air in." He denies having fever or chills but mentions that he has had a dry cough for the past three days. Otherwise, he has no symptoms. His medications include chlorpropamide (an oral hypoglycemic) and hydrochlorothiazide.

Dr. Ellsworth completes the history and physical exam and draws some blood for laboratory tests. It is 2 AM when she leaves Mr. Friend and writes his admission orders. She quickly checks the hospital formulary for dosage, but in prescribing medications, she writes that the patient should receive chlorpromazine (a major tranquilizer) instead of chlorpropamide.

Over the weekend, Mr. Friend's respiratory status improves markedly. Late Sunday evening, as Dr. Ellsworth is preparing her presentation of the weekend admissions for the Monday chief of service rounds, she reviews Mr. Friend's medication list and notices her prescription error. She immediately goes to check on the patient, who is alert and well without symptoms. Dr. Ellsworth asks the nurse to do a finger stick to assess Mr. Friend's blood glucose level and to draw blood for a stat glucose test. The finger stick indicates a glucose level of 137. The stat glucose level is 150.

Dr. Ellsworth is relieved. Fortunately, her error has not harmed Mr. Friend. But now she must deal with a more difficult problem: whether to disclose her error to Dr. Rhys, the chief of service. Should she disclose the confusion over the name of the medication to the patient? Is she ethically responsible to disclose her error, even though no harm resulted from it?

———⟫⬦⟪———

COMMENTARY

When should physicians disclose errors to patients and colleagues? This case study considers the issue in the context of training because the way in which physicians handle errors made during training has direct bearing on how they will handle mistakes made during the course of their careers.

Errors are inherent to the practice of medicine. They arise from medical uncertainty about diagnosis and about the risks and benefits of treatments. The environment in which decisions are made is also conducive to mistakes: Decisions often must be made quickly, with limited knowledge; many decisions affecting different patients must be made virtually simultaneously; and medical care, especially in the hospital setting, now involves many steps and people, all of whom must be well coordinated and integrated to deliver high-quality care. As the system of care becomes more complex, the probability for error increases.

Studies have examined the frequency and severity of errors, especially in the training setting (1, 2). In one study, nearly all interns reported having made a mistake that had serious consequences for patients (1). While the coping and socialization processes surrounding medical mistakes have been the subject of several studies (2–7), relatively little information exists on the criteria clinicians apply when they decide whether to disclose errors to their patients, colleagues, or supervising physicians. Evidence suggests that in more than half of the cases, residents do not discuss their mistakes with their attendings (1).

The typical mechanisms that physicians use for facing their mistakes have been well described (2). Initially, physicians use denial—the process by which errors are justified because medicine is an "art" as much as a science and because there are often no right or wrong answers, only differences of opinion. Then they use discounting—the process by which the responsibility for errors is assigned to external agents: They may blame the system, their superiors for having faltered despite their greater degree of experience, the disease process, the inadequacies of scientific knowledge, or the patient. Physicians may also use distancing—because everyone makes mistakes, personal responsibility is lessened. Mistakes can then be accepted as natural and understandable, and guilt can be assuaged: "I did everything I could; we all make errors. You can't know it all" (2).

Unfortunately, most of these coping mechanisms do not foster the principles of learning or of continuous improvement that ultimately lead to better patient care. One study clearly demonstrated that such responses to mistakes—responses that often are fostered by the graduate medical education socialization process—isolate the trainees (2). These physicians come to believe that because they are solely responsible for their actions, they should also be their own and "worst" judge, which leads them to discount attempts by others to insert them into a system of accountability. Thus, most trainees out of principles of self-reliance choose not to disclose errors to their professional colleagues or administrative superiors.

In our case, Dr. Ellsworth has discovered her prescription error and corrected it in a timely fashion. The patient suffered no harm from the mistake. Does Dr. Ellsworth have further responsibilities in this situation? Does she have an ethical obligation to report the mistake to Mr. Friend or Dr. Rhys, the attending physician of record?

Most codes of ethics are silent when it comes to physicians' obligations to report errors to patients. The Canadian Medical Association and the American Medical Association codes of ethics do not directly address the duty to disclose errors to patients (8). The latest edition of the American College of Physicians *Ethics Manual*, on the other hand, gives general guidance: ". . . physicians should disclose to patients information about procedural or judgment errors made in the course of care, if such information significantly affects the care of the patient. Errors do not necessarily constitute improper, negligent, or unethical behavior" (9).

Available data suggest that in most cases physicians are reluctant to tell patients about mistakes. In one study of internal medicine house officers, only 24% told the patient or the family about mistakes affecting them (1). In a 1984 study, 78 out of 83 trainees interviewed did not believe that revealing errors to patients or families was an option they would consider (2).

The *Ethics Manual* is clear about the responsibilities of physicians in training to "acknowledge their limitations and ask for help or supervision from their attending physicians, chiefs of service, or consultants when concerns arise about patient care. . . . Residents must keep the attending physicians informed about each patient's hospital course and treatment plan" (9).

As Dr. Ellsworth decides what to do, she considers the consequences of disclosure and begins to weigh the benefits and harms to herself, personally and professionally, and to her patient. She is tempted not to tell Mr. Friend because she believes that this could result in more harm than good. The disclosure would make no difference to his well-being, as she had already made sure he was not harmed by the error. She reasons that he could be distressed to learn that an error occurred and that he might lose confidence in the quality of care provided by her and the hospital. Indeed, trivial errors happen in the hospital setting and do not necessarily reflect negligence.

But not disclosing the error also carries the risk for harm to the patient. Mr. Friend could discover the error on his own or learn of it from a nurse. He then would have cause to doubt the integrity of the professionals involved in his care, which might jeopardize the trust essential to the physician–patient relationship. Without this trust, communication between physician and patient falters, and a harmful, adversarial relationship often ensues. Open communication is best for addressing the fear of litigation, given that the breakdown or absence of an ongoing relationship between patient and physician increases the risk for legal suits.

Given these risks, in general, all relevant information should be disclosed to allow patients to participate fully in decisions about their care. This information includes disclosure of errors that significantly affect care. Although more discretion can be exercised in disclosing trivial errors (for example, a one-time substitution of a low-fat diet for a normal one or an extra urine sample collected because of a laboratory accident), in most cases an honest discussion with the patient can and should ensue.

As a rule, physicians should begin with the premise that all errors be revealed, unless good reasons exist to do otherwise. These reasons should relate to the circumstances and preferences of each patient, as gauged by the physician in the context of an established physician–patient relationship. For example, it might be appropriate to withhold knowledge of a trivial error from a patient who prefers not to hear most clinical details and only wants the big picture; it might also be acceptable in the case of a patient in an extremely fragile physical or emotional state. However, because truth telling is fundamental to the patient–physician relationship, the burden of proof for nondisclosure should remain great, with well-defined reasons based on the physician's best clinical judgment.

Dr. Ellsworth is reluctant to tell Dr. Rhys of her error because she is afraid that disclosure will affect her reputation among her colleagues and might even initiate embarrassing reviews of her performance, which could then compromise her competitiveness when she applies for a fellowship next year. Since the error did not hurt the patient, she figures that she would do no harm by not telling. She reasons that as long as she remains self-critical and learns from this mistake to be more careful when prescribing medications, she may have fulfilled her responsibility.

On the other hand, she feels uncomfortable with keeping this secret. By failing to reveal a mistake, even one without any consequence for patient outcome, she is hiding important information about the management course from the physician who is ultimately responsible for Mr. Friend's care.

She is also contributing to an environment in which mistakes are kept secret and neglecting the opportunity for everyone to learn from mistakes and to improve the quality of care. Although Dr. Ellsworth made the prescription error, others in the delivery loop failed to identify the error and prevent it. The attending did not thoroughly review the orders or the medication sheets, and the nursing staff failed to notice that the medications ordered differed from the ones that the patient was taking at the time of admission. Nor did the pharmacists notice or question the change in medication. This error could provide an opportunity to apply the principles of quality improvement by adopting a system-based approach to problem solving.

Dr. Ellsworth also acknowledges that her error may have important implications for the patient's future management. In the face of an acute stressor, Mr. Friend did well without his hypoglycemic medication and may not need this drug at all. But no one will know this unless Dr. Ellsworth tells Dr. Rhys about her mistake. Dr. Rhys is ultimately accountable for the patient's care. He must trust that house staff is completely honest about all aspects of the patient's course because he needs this knowledge to make informed and clinically responsible management decisions.

Clinical training is a time when newly acquired diagnostic and therapeutic skills are put into practice. The theory of medicine, acquired in the preceding nonclinical years, is finally applied to the real world of patient care, and the uncertainties of medicine are discovered. As with any new endeavor, some mistakes will occur. They may be caused by errors of judgment, lack of knowledge or technical skills, or the pressures of the practice environment.

Errors may result when communication breaks down among the many individuals involved in delivering care, if the system of care has inefficiencies or just by chance. Some errors are unavoidable or unpredictable. No matter what the cause or severity of the error, or its consequences for the patient's outcome, the training environment should encourage learning and continuous improvement because early experiences are likely to set the tone for how physicians will deal with errors throughout their careers.

Medical practice, during both the training period and the much longer post-training period, is fraught with the possibility of making errors. The knowledge gained from these errors is essential to improve the quality of one's practice. Improvement can only happen if the climate promotes free exchange of information and if errors are dealt with in a constructive rather than purely punitive fashion. In one study of house officers' response to mistakes, only 54% discussed serious errors with their attending (1). Eighty-eight percent reported talking about an error with another colleague in a nonsupervisory role, and 5% told no one about it.

The study also showed that 90% of the reported errors resulted in serious adverse outcomes—physical discomfort, emotional distress, additional therapy or procedures, or prolonged hospital stay. In 31% of the reported cases, the patient died. In the same study, house officers were also more likely to report constructive changes in their practice of medicine if they accepted responsibility for the mistake and discussed it with their attending.

Returning to our case, we believe that Dr. Ellsworth should disclose her error, no matter how trivial, to her attending physician. They could then discuss the case, assess how the error affected management and outcome, and decide whether to disclose it to the patient. Mistakes that significantly affect care should always be disclosed to the patient.

As a profession, we must bring the issue of medical errors out in the open. We need to foster an environment in which physicians and patients acknowledge that errors happen and recognize that we all can and should learn from them. Just as the physician-in-training has a responsibility to discuss any mistakes with the attending of record, the attending also has the responsibility to encourage such discussions and to create a valuable learning experience.

We should strive to create an atmosphere in which errors can be resolved in an ethical and responsible manner. Truth telling is essential to improving medical practice and to professional relationships among physicians. It forms the cornerstone of trust between physicians and patients. As a general rule, lying or omitting information undermines these relationships and the public's trust in the medical profession. Disclosing an error to a colleague or patient may cause short-term discomfort, tension, or even ridicule; nevertheless, its long-term benefits for the physician who erred, for the patient, and for the environment in which other health professionals deliver care far outweigh the risks of secrecy.

REFERENCES

1. Wu AW, Folkman S, McPhee S, Lo B. Do house officers learn from their mistakes? JAMA. 1991;265:2089-94.
2. Mizrahi T. Managing medical mistakes: ideology, insularity and accountability among internists-in-training. Soc Sci Med. 1984;19:135-46.
3. Novack DH, Detering BJ, Arnold R, Forrow L, Ladinsky M, Pezzullo JC. Physicians' attitudes toward using deception to resolve difficult ethical problems. JAMA. 1989;261:2980-5.
4. Hilfiker D. Sounding board: facing our mistakes. N Engl J Med. 1984;310:118-22.
5. Christensen JF, Levinson W, Dunn P. The heart of darkness: the impact of perceived mistakes on physicians. J Gen Intern Med. 1992;7:424-31.
6. Light D. Uncertainty and control in professional training. J Health Soc Behav. 1979;20:310-22.
7. Bosk CL. Forgive and Remember: Managing Medical Failure. Chicago: University of Chicago Press; 1979.
8. Warner E. Telling patients about medical negligence. Can Med Assoc J. 1983;129:366-8.

9. American College of Physicians. American College of Physicians Ethics Manual. Third edition. Ann Intern Med. 1992;117:947-60.

Annotated Bibliography

Novack DH, Detering BJ, Arnold R, Forrow L, Ladinsky M, Pezzullo JC. Physicians' attitudes toward using deception to resolve difficult ethical problems. JAMA. 1989;261:2980-5.

In response to case scenarios and general questions about attitudes and current practices, most physicians said they would engage in deception of insurers, patients, and families based on potential health care consequences, patient welfare, and the protection of confidentiality.

Wu AW, Folkman S, McPhee S, Lo B. Do house officers learn from their mistakes? JAMA. 1991;265:2089-94.

Internal medicine house officers who acknowledged, accepted responsibility for, and discussed their mistakes were more likely to make constructive changes in their practice.

Part IV

The Business of Medicine: Effects on the Patient–Physician Relationship

The practice of medicine does not take place in a vacuum. It occurs within a context—the health care system—and within our unique American culture.

Economic issues have implications for the delivery of care. Two issues are dealt with here. Financial incentives and their potential influence on clinical decision making in both managed care and fee-for-service indemnity settings are considered in Chapter 14, whereas Chapter 15 looks at issues raised by the role the drug industry has played in the financial support of continuing medical education activities, interactions between the drug industry and medicine, and potential effects of this interaction on patient care.

14

Financial Incentives and Physician Decision Making

Commentary by LOIS SNYDER, JD
Case History by ALAN L. HILLMAN, MD, MBA, FACP

CASE HISTORY

Ted and Ned are 46-year-old, asymptomatic, sedentary identical twins. Both are executives in local corporations. Former smokers—both smoked about one-half pack per day from their late teens to their early thirties, when they quit as a New Year's resolution—they have been generally healthy except for mild obesity, secondary to many executive lunches. As a New Year's resolution for 1990, Ted and Ned agree to join a local gym to "tone up" and get back in shape. Both had been college athletes. The gym requires a note from

Continued

each man's doctor before starting the exercise program, but no specific tests were mandated.

Ted had enrolled in GreatCare, an independent practice association (IPA)-model HMO, because he liked the "comprehensive care" concept, including an emphasis on prevention and wellness. He also valued the idea of no out-of-pocket health care costs other than the premium deducted from his paycheck. Because the HMO is an IPA-model, in which the HMO contracts with independent providers in private practice, Ted was able to select a local physician about whom he had heard good things.

Unbeknownst to Ted, his physician had agreed to certain contractual arrangements with the HMO. Among them were a 15% discount on his usual fees and an additional 15% withholding. The HMO would return the 15% withholding to the physician only if his referral account for specialist services and laboratory tests had a surplus at the end of the year. If the referral account had a surplus, the physician would get his withheld funds and a bonus equal to half of his share of any surplus in the referral pool. The HMO, which had grouped Ted's physician with four others in his community as a risk pool, provided him with the names, addresses, and telephone numbers of these other physicians and encouraged him to contact the group to "discuss the use of referral funds from their aggregate pool."

Ned, on the other hand, had selected traditional indemnity fee-for-service health care insurance, and his premiums and out-of-pocket payments were higher than Ted's. Ned felt that retaining complete freedom of choice with respect to doctors was important, despite the somewhat higher overall costs. As is usual in traditional fee-for-service health care, Ned's doctor is paid for each patient visit and every service performed.

Ted and Ned met at the gym for their first joint workout. Ned mentioned that his physician would not write a note for him to start the program without first

performing an electrocardiogram and exercise tolerance test (the results of which were normal). Ned takes
some pride in what he considers to be his doctor's comprehensive approach to his health care and the extra
attention he got for clearance for the exercise program.
Ted wants to know why *his* doctor did not order these
tests. After some thought, Ned begins to wonder if the
expensive and time-consuming tests he received really
were needed. Both brothers are confused.

———⟫•◇•⟪———

COMMENTARY

The physician's primary obligations are to the patient, not to the system under which he or she provides care and certainly not to the
physician's own pocketbook. Following the ethical course under
medically clear circumstances is obviously easiest: An exercise tolerance test would be medically unnecessary for a 20-year-old female
college athlete with no risk factors who is about to join a gym.

Most situations require physician judgment as to whether an
intervention or test is appropriate for a given patient. The objectivity of physician discretion must not be allowed to be affected by
external forces.

The American College of Physicians *Ethics Manual* says, "The
welfare of the patient must at all times be paramount, and the physician must insist that the medically appropriate level of care takes
primacy over fiscal considerations. . . . The guiding principle should
always be care consistent with humanistic, scientific, and efficient
medicine. . . . In the final analysis, no external factors should interfere with the dedication of the physician to provide optimal care for
his or her patient" (1).

In addition to obvious influences on behavior, physicians must be
aware of more subtle influences that could affect judgment when the
best clinical decision for a patient is unclear; for example, in the fee-
for-service setting, a physician may too quickly recommend a test or
procedure, whereas the HMO physician may adopt a wait-and-see
approach for too long (2).

The patient–physician relationship necessarily involves unequal partners. Vulnerable patients entrust their health and lives to physicians, the keepers and communicators of medical knowledge. Patients have the right to make informed decisions about their care. But physicians have the power to influence decision making.

With fee-for-service, more tests mean more fees. Physicians must be aware of and seek to avoid the "more is better" philosophy that this setting might implicitly encourage. Some commentators have said that potential conflict is easier for the patient to see in this setting; patients know that the more the doctor does, the more he gets paid. The patient's ability to verify the medical need for a service by getting a second opinion can serve as a check on physician behavior (3).

Such verification of need is certainly an option when the patient is considering a major operation, but Ned has no reason to question his doctor's judgment that exercise testing is required to evaluate whether he can join the gym. And even if the second opinion "check" theory were applicable more often, it would not convert ethically unacceptable behavior into ethically acceptable behavior.

In the HMO setting, if a medically needed service is denied because incentives distort physician judgment rather than merely encourage cost-effective care, the patient will probably not know it. Here, there has been no discourse between physician and patient. In the fee-for-service context, something affirmative has to happen before the physician profits—the physician must propose the service and do the test. If the physician refers the patient elsewhere and if something other than appropriate care motivates the referral, these actions raise issues ranging from fee splitting to unnecessary referrals.

In the HMO setting, the patient may not know a type of care is being omitted. Some patients may question what they see as a lack of care, for example, if they expected to have a test or receive a prescription, but others may not know what care is missing.

A number of lawsuits naming HMOs as defendants are now making their way through the courts. Plaintiffs have alleged that HMO incentive systems, which had not been disclosed to them upon their joining, compromised the independent judgment of primary physicians and resulted in poor health care services. Physicians can themselves end up as defendants. In the fee-for-service setting, fear of lawsuits has been cited as the basis for so-called "defensive medicine," but this fear does not justify providing unnecessary care. The practice and documentation of medically appropriate care remain the best defense in a medical malpractice action. The threat of lawsuits should no more affect care than clinical judgment should be distorted by financial incentives.

In a fee-for-service practice, a physician may consciously or unconsciously over-test. In using tests appropriately, physicians should look not only at the immediate cost of a test but should also consider the additional expenses that can mount in following up a false-positive result. Also important are the potential medical complications in the performance of the original test or follow-up and the anxiety patients may suffer while waiting to find out if they actually have the disease or condition. These are reasons that the American College of Physicians and others have been developing guidelines for the use of common tests in screening, case-finding, diagnosis, and management of disease.

However, a physician attempting to care for Ted or Ned according to the American College of Physicians's medical necessity guidelines on "Screening for Asymptomatic Coronary Artery Disease: Exercise Stress Testing" (4) and on "Screening for Asymptomatic CAD: The Resting Electrocardiogram" (4) would be in a gray zone and would have to rely on individual judgment.

The exercise stress testing guidelines state:

> Exercise testing is not recommended as a routine screening procedure in adults with no evidence of coronary heart disease and no risk factors. . . . Some asymptomatic persons may have particular reasons to consider exercise stress testing for coronary artery disease. Some persons are especially likely to have the disease because of increased age, male gender, and at least one other risk factor (family history of CAD, cigarette smoking, diabetes mellitus, systolic blood pressure greater than 140 mm Hg, hypercholesterolemia, or a cholesterol to HDL ratio of more than 6.0). Other persons who should be tested are those who have an occu-

pation that puts others at risk (for example, bus drivers or airline pilots) or are sedentary and about to begin a program of physical conditioning. There is insufficient evidence to make a strong recommendation for or against use of routine stress testing in these groups.

Similarly, the resting electrocardiogram guidelines list the above risk factors for coronary artery disease and state: "The resting ECG [electrocardiogram] is not recommended as a routine practice in people who are under age 65 and do not have evidence for cardiovascular disease or its risk factors. However, it may be appropriate in selected patients, especially in situations where the published evidence is not decisive."

The fact that the brothers are former cigarette smokers could put them at increased risk for coronary artery disease, but this possibility is not as clear-cut as it would be for current smokers or those who smoked several packs per day or had quit more recently. The fact that both patients are sedentary and mildly obese and the nature of the exercise program each is about to start are additional considerations for the physicians to evaluate. Decision making is also affected by variation in the information elicited by different physicians in the history and physical examination. Styles of diagnosis and management, personalities, and the patients' needs and preferences all can affect medical choices.

As long as these and other medical factors were the reasons for the decisions about testing, then the best interest of each patient is motivating each physician. As it turns out, each doctor's income was enhanced because the fee-for-service physician performed the tests on Ned, while the HMO doctor, whose take-home pay could be reduced had he ordered the tests, did not order them for Ted.

Finally, the comparison of the care they received has left both Ned and Ted somewhat confused. Patients need to be able to have confidence in the care they receive and must always be fully informed about medical care. Given the circumstances, Ted's physician probably did not need to explain why he omitted tests he felt were not medically indicated (unless the patient had asked about it specifically), although he should explain his reasoning fully when and if

Ted raises the issue at his next visit. Likewise, Ned's physician may need to go into greater detail about his decisions at Ned's request. Decisions that patients perceive as conflicts of interest on the part of their physician can undermine the patient–physician relationship.

Physicians have an ethical duty to be aware of the financial incentives of the system in which they practice and the possibility of obvious and subtle influences. Disclosing financial incentives and interests might provide patients with needed information, although this will not necessarily remedy conflicts. Little has been written about the mechanics of disclosure—for example, how and what information should be presented and what oversight measures are needed to ensure compliance (5).

Disclosure might range from physician statements about ownership interests in a laboratory or other health care entity to which the physician refers patients to explanations of the incentives of particular practice settings. Physicians are not relieved of their obligation to serve the best interests of their patients, however, whether or not they or the organizations for which they work disclose the relevant financial incentives under which they practice medicine.

REFERENCES

1. American College of Physicians. American College of Physicians Ethics Manual. Ann Intern Med. 1989;111:245-52, 327-35.
2. Hillman A. Health maintenance organizations, financial incentives, and physicians' judgments. Ann Intern Med. 1990;112:891-3.
3. Morreim H. Conflicts of interest: profits and problems in physician referrals. JAMA. 1989;262:390-4.
4. Eddy DM. Common screening tests. Philadelphia: American College of Physicians, 1991.
5. Rodwin M. Physicians' conflicts of interest: the limitations of disclosure. N Engl J Med. 1989;321:1405-8.

ANNOTATED BIBLIOGRAPHY

Council on Ethical and Judicial Affairs, American Medical Association. Ethical issues in managed care. JAMA. 1995;273:330-5.

The American Medical Association's guidelines about ethics under managed care. Looks at conflicts among patients, conflicts between physician and patient, patient responsibility, and bedside rationing.

Igelhart JK. Efforts to address the problem of physician self-referral. N Engl J Med. 1991;325:1820-4.

> Examines at physician business practices that raise concerns and the governmental response—self-referral bans and the development of "safe harbors" for business arrangements that would not violate the Medicare-Medicaid anti-kickback statutes and regulations.

Rodwin MA. Conflicts in managed care. N Engl J Med. 1995;332:604-7.

> Describes a "conflict" model of managed care, its ethical and legal implications, and methods for dealing with the conflicts.

Thompson DF. Understanding financial conflicts of interest. N Engl J Med. 1993;329:573-6.

> Defines conflict of interest broadly; reviews potential standards for assessing conflicts and remedies, including individual provider discretion, professional and governmental regulation, and disclosure; and calls for clear guidelines for avoiding conflicts.

Wolf SM. Health care reform and the future of physician ethics. Hastings Cent Rep. 1994;24:28-41.

> Discusses ethical tensions inherent in reform models and in efforts at cost-consciousness and cost-containment; analyzes proposals for clarifying physician obligations and proposes the development of a new ethics of institutions.

15

Pharmaceutical Industry Support of Continuing Medical Education

Commentaries by JANET WEINER, MPH, LOIS SNYDER, JD, KATHLEEN L. EGAN, PhD, **and** FRANK DAVIDOFF, MD, FACP
Case History by JANET WEINER, MPH, **and** LOIS SNYDER, JD

CASE HISTORY

Dr. Sira Assad is a general internist practicing in a working-class neighborhood of a small city. At the end of a busy day, she emerges from the examination room in great frustration after seeing a long-time patient, Ms. Bertha Lake. Ms. Lake, a 67-year-old woman with hypertension, follows Dr. Assad slowly to her office.

"Ms. Lake, you need to be taking this medication every day. Not every other day, not half the dosage.

Continued

Your blood pressure is 185/100, even higher than it was last month."

Ms. Lake tells of her ongoing concerns and anxiety about her finances. "But Dr. Assad, I can't afford that stuff. I live on a fixed income, and the pills cost $70 a month. Medicare doesn't cover them. Can't we go with something cheaper?"

Dr. Assad remembers that she tried other less expensive drugs, but they did not adequately control Ms. Lake's blood pressure. Dr. Assad feels helpless. "Here are some free samples . . . they'll tide you over until you can find a way to pay for the drug. It's very important to get back on it and stay on it . . . " Dr. Assad gives Ms. Lake the rest of the samples left by the drug company representative (a three-week supply) and worries about what will happen when they run out. She gives her patient a new prescription and a return appointment and tells her to call if she cannot fill the prescription.

After Ms. Lake leaves, Dr. Assad calls the drug representative to ask for more samples. The drug rep says that he cannot replenish her supply because he did so just two days before. Dr. Assad asks whether the company has a program for supplying indigent patients with drugs at no or reduced cost; the rep replies that the company does not have a program in place but is in the process of devising one.

The next morning, after visiting her patients at the hospital, Dr. Assad gets a call from the hospital's director of medical education, Dr. Gabriel Fowler. Like Dr. Assad, Dr. Fowler is a busy private practitioner. Serving as chair of the medical education committee is part of his "pay back" to the hospital. Dr. Fowler takes his responsibilities as director quite seriously and has spent many hours in the last few months planning a continuing medical education (CME) program to update primary care physicians on cardiovascular disease. He has procured an educational grant from a drug company for the program and has insisted on maintaining control of the program content and the speakers invited. His mission today is to spread the word to his colleagues and urge them to register for the program.

Dr. Assad listens as Dr. Fowler reminds her about the deadline to register for this full-day program to be held at a convenient local hotel. Dr. Assad, after hearing about the topics and faculty, signs up. The program has no registration fee and includes a full dinner.

A few weeks later, Dr. Assad is listening to an excellent lecture in the CME program when her beeper goes off. Ms. Lake has called, scared and wanting to know if she should go to the hospital. Suddenly, she has found that she cannot speak clearly and her right hand is clumsy. Her face feels funny and looks "off balance" in the mirror. Thoughts race through Dr. Assad's mind: Is this an accomplished stroke or a transient ischemic attack? Is this happening because Ms. Lake has just run out of medication? Or is Ms. Lake paying the price for inadequate control of her blood pressure over time?

On the way to meet her patient at the emergency room, Dr. Assad looks at the program materials in her hands and realizes that the pharmaceutical company supporter of the CME program produces the drug that Ms. Lake cannot afford. She suddenly feels confused and resentful. How much cheaper would the drug be if the company did not spend so much on glossy advertisements, brochures, handouts, pens, samples, and fancy CME dinners? Why are drug reps milling around the reception area at the CME conference? Why is her hospital accepting this kind of largess? Is she being taken advantage of? Is her patient paying, indirectly, for the amenities of this meeting?

At the hospital the next day, Dr. Assad runs into Dr. Fowler and voices her discomfort with the circumstances of the meeting. She is surprised when Dr. Fowler becomes impatient.

"How do you expect a small hospital to pay for such a high-quality meeting?" he asked. "You know how expensive it is to print and mail brochures, to bring in faculty from leading academic medical centers, to rent the space and provide decent meals. The companies want to pay for it, and good CME is hard to find near home. You should be glad we can arrange it!"

Dr. Assad is not convinced. When it is her turn to direct medical education at the hospital, she wonders, will she do things differently?

⟹◈⟸

DR. ASSAD'S COMMENTARY

In her proper role as an advocate for her patient, Dr. Assad is questioning the actions of both the pharmaceutical industry and the medical profession within a system that fails to guarantee that medically necessary drugs will be affordable for all people. She is making connections between seemingly unconnected events in her professional life that may be contributing to a medically and ethically unacceptable outcome for her patient.

For money to stand in the way of Ms. Lake's ability to obtain a needed drug is morally unacceptable. And yet this is a reality for her and many other patients. Some would argue that this problem is a result of gaps in insurance coverage, while others argue that the high price of drugs is primarily to blame. Our health care system is flawed on both counts; high prices probably contribute to the widening gaps in insurance, and both factors combine to create the economic and moral dilemma we face.

In 1988 (the most recent year for which comparative figures were available), retail spending for prescription drugs amounted to $27.1 billion, 56% of which was paid for out of pocket by consumers (1). The elderly, who constituted 12% of the total population in 1988, accounted for 35% of prescription drug expenditures (1). Meanwhile, 16 pharmaceutical companies surveyed by the Senate (2) spent $85.9 million in 1988 sponsoring 34,688 scientific symposia. In the same year, the pharmaceutical industry was estimated to spend about $200 million a year on medical education (as distinct from promotional activities) (3). In general, the industry is estimated to spend probably more than $10 billion a year on promotion, which exceeds their spending on research by $1 billion (4). Overall, the drug industry spends about 24% of its sales revenue on promotion (2).

Promotion or Education?

The ethics of industry-supported CME have mostly focused on the distinction between promotion and education, emphasizing the need to resist promotional bias and maintain the scientific integrity of the programs. The importance of CME providers maintaining control of the content of educational programs has been underscored most recently by the Food and Drug Administration (FDA) (5), but also by the American Medical Association (AMA) (6), the American College of Physicians (3), and many others. However, existing ethical guidelines are noticeably silent on the question of the physician's role in influencing the affordability of prescription drugs. Beyond being cost-conscious and prescribing only medically necessary drugs, does the physician have an obligation to influence the broader forces that result in drug prices beyond the means of many patients?

Dr. Assad is aware that many drug companies offer indigent patient programs. In a 1992 directory published by the Pharmaceutical Manufacturers Association, 59 companies listed indigent programs covering a varying number of drugs and having different eligibility requirements (7). Dr. Assad has used this service in the past, and a few of her poor patients have benefited. But from experience, she knows that these programs often have cumbersome paperwork requirements for certifying eligibility and for continuous recertification and often do not serve people who are just beyond the poverty level. She is convinced that these programs, although they respond compassionately to some people in desperate need, do not meet the needs of many people who cannot afford expensive medications.

Dr. Assad has noted that the pharmaceutical companies spend considerable funds on physicians and physician groups. The money is spent on detailing, distribution of free samples, advertising (including promotional booths and materials at educational functions), and direct support for educational activities. The companies set the prices of their drugs, and these pricing decisions have led to a relatively high level of industry profits, according to some analysts (8, 9). Given these business decisions, it is not unreasonable to conclude that pharmaceutical companies pass the cost of their relationships with the medical profession on to consumers through inflated prices.

On the other hand, lessening support of CME does not automatically mean that drug prices will be lower. Continuing medical education providers have no control over the funds that they refuse and therefore, on a practical level, cannot ensure that drugs will become more affordable for patients. Further, both patients and physicians may lose the benefits derived from this spending, for example, quality CME programs and free samples for patients.

The controversy has led several commentators to question the need for the industry's support of CME. "The pharmaceutical industry must promote and sell its products. Medical education must educate and avoid promotion. We are in a quandary of our own making because we have decided that we cannot afford to educate ourselves without this industry's support" (10).

Another physician, Dr. Douglas Waud, writes, "I believe physicians can buy books and attend meetings without fear of landing in the poorhouse" (11). He maintains that subsidies for meetings are "bribes" that free up physicians' own money for other purposes. Because this money comes out of the pockets of patients, Dr. Waud finds it "at odds with the physician's responsibility to act in the best interests of the patient" (11).

And what about the free samples that Dr. Assad gave to Ms. Lake? She has reason to question the benefits of this aspect of pharmaceutical promotion as well. Manufacturers distributed 2.4 billion samples in 1988 (2), yet little published information exists on the clinical use of sample medications. A recent study concluded that although most medications dispensed were given to patients, approximately one third of the value of the medications either went to physicians and their families or had an unknown destination (12). The authors found a high association between sample dispensing and simultaneous prescribing of the same brand-name drug, which supports the contention that sampling influences physicians' prescribing habits. Although this influence might not be the decisive factor for Dr. Assad and Ms. Lake in our case study, the overall effect on prescribing patterns cannot be ignored. If this effect is combined with evidence that most physicians do not know the actual prices of drugs (13), it is easy to see how samples may actually contribute to higher out-of-pocket drug costs for patients.

Are physicians prepared to forgo CME subsidies, drug samples, and other amenities provided by the pharmaceutical industry? If so, can physicians at the same time pressure the pharmaceutical companies to lower their prices? The answers to both questions are not clear. However, Dr. Assad will surely find the answers if she attempts to conduct CME programs without industry support. Given the social, medical, and economic costs to patients, efforts to minimize the medical profession's reliance on pharmaceutical industry support are worth a try.

DR. FOWLER'S COMMENTARY

Dr. Fowler is somewhat taken aback by Dr. Assad's reaction to the meeting. Is she trying to say that pharmaceutical industry support of CME should be banned? He does not agree. For him, the issue is not whether there should be any relationship between the drug industry and physicians but rather how to define that relationship for the good of patients. "A responsible and productive alliance between the medical profession and the pharmaceutical industry is unquestionably beneficial to medical progress . . . partnered activities offer important opportunities to impartially advance the state of medical practice and thus improve patient care" (3).

As director of medical education, Dr. Fowler has closely followed issues on the ethics of industry-supported CME and industry gifts to doctors, including the development of guidelines by the FDA, the Accreditation Council for Continuing Medical Education (14), the American Medical Association, the Pharmaceutical Manufacturers Association (15), the American College of Physicians, and others. For these groups and for Dr. Fowler, the ethical issues surrounding CME are about distinguishing between education and promotion and maintaining the scientific integrity of programs.

Medical education and scientific exchange are important endeavors that lead to improved patient care. Promotion of particular products, on the other hand, should be labeled as such and regulated; subtle or disguised promotion that introduces bias into supposedly objective publications and programs should be eliminated. Physicians have an ethical obligation to their patients, to the profession, and to society to preserve the objectivity of clinical judgment and avoid even the appearance of outside influences. They must confront issues of potential bias in evaluating medical information whatever the source, be it academic, professional, or commercial.

In the CME context, Dr. Fowler believes that physicians must be especially sensitive to the need to eliminate, or at a minimum to control, potential bias in any commercial presentation of medical information. To that end, he has scrupulously followed the guidelines of the groups noted above and maintained complete control over program content and faculty selection. When the drug company approached him with available funds, he accepted on the condition that he and his colleagues be in control of topic and faculty selection.

They settled on a comprehensive update on cardiovascular disease, a topic of many dimensions, great relevance in the community, and wide appeal to the medical staff. Speakers were required to disclose any financial or other interests that might affect their presentation. The drug company had no role in the course budget, honoraria payment, or selection of who attended the program. Company funding was disclosed. Drug reps and promotional materials were not permitted in or near the meeting room. Dr. Fowler considers the hospitality provided to be modest. He feels safe in declaring that the program was not biased by the source of funding.

Would Prices Change?

So why is Dr. Assad so concerned, he wonders? Does she believe that decreasing or ending pharmaceutical industry support for CME will automatically mean that drug prices will be lower? The amount of money spent on CME by industry ($200 million) does not even begin to compare with what pharmaceutical companies spend collectively on promotion in the United States—some $10 billion a year (16). And as a percentage of the $27 billion in retail spending on prescription drugs, $200 million amounts to less than 1%.

Had he refused the funds, the company likely would have just gone to another hospital. This event would have put Dr. Fowler's medical staff, for whom he is charged with providing quality CME, at a disadvantage. The patients, who benefit from their doctors' continuing education, would also lose out. Could they have put on a program of this quality with their own resources? Should they?

The issue of drug prices must be seen in the larger context of universal access to health care. Are physicians obligated to influence the broader forces that result in drug prices beyond the means of patients? Dr. Fowler believes the answer is yes—to the extent that physicians must be advocates for public health, especially within the current debate about health care reform. For Dr. Fowler, though, the direct care of patients is the ethical issue and one that physicians can do something about. But many physicians do not even accept Medicare or Medicaid patients into their practices, let alone uninsured people. "What about their care?" he remembers asking during a heated discussion with a colleague. Ethics, it seems to Dr. Fowler, begin at home—in the physician's office.

On further reflection, Dr. Fowler is reminded of the reaction of many physicians when medical groups and others first started issuing guidelines for physician–pharmaceutical relations. No group had proposed that pharmaceutical support be branded as unethical per se and banned. Instead, guidelines were suggested to help define and ensure ethical relations and behavior. Even so, many physicians felt that they were being treated as though they were "guilty until proven innocent." Julian Berman, MD, of Coral Springs, Florida, wrote:

> I am not at an academic medical center. The medical education available to me without leaving the office for a week to travel . . . consists of pharmaceutical company–sponsored lectures given by experts at our local hospitals and restaurants and weekend meetings in pleasant surroundings that feature nationally known speakers . . . I am generally sick and tired of having my ethical sense denigrated by editors and academics who do not know me, how I

make my decisions, or for that matter, what decisions I make. To answer the question posed in the American College of Physicians position paper (3), I would not mind at all if my arrangements with the pharmaceutical industry were generally known (17).

Dr. Berman was referring to the Royal College of Physicians guideline, "Would I be willing to have this arrangement generally known?" which was adopted by the American College of Physicians along with the query, "What would the public or my patients think of this arrangement?" (18). Regarding the recent educational conference and industry support of CME in general, Dr. Fowler feels comfortable with his answers to these questions.

REFERENCES

1. Office of National Cost Estimates. National health expenditures, 1988. Health Care Financing Review. 1990;11:1-54.
2. U.S. Senate, Committee on Labor and Human Resources. Advertising, marketing, and promotional practices of the pharmaceutical industry, hearing Dec. 11 and 12, 1990. Washington, D.C.: U.S. Government Printing Office; 1991.
3. American College of Physicians. Physicians and the pharmaceutical industry. Ann Intern Med. 1990;112:624-6.
4. New York Times, 21 Feb. 1993, p. 1 et seq.
5. Food and Drug Administration. Draft policy statement on industry-supported scientific and educational activities [docket no. 92N-0434]. Federal Register, 27 Nov. 1992.
6. Council on Ethical and Judicial Affairs. Gifts to physicians from industry. JAMA. 1991;265:501.
7. Pharmaceutical Manufacturers Association. 1992 Directory of Prescription Drug Indigent Programs (advertisement). American Medical News, 24-31 Aug. 1992, pp. 21-4.
8. U.S. General Accounting Office. Prescription Drugs—Companies Typically Charge More in the United States Than in Canada. Washington, D.C.: General Accounting Office; September 1992. Publication no. GAO/HRD-92-110.
9. Office of Technology Assessment. Pharmaceutical R&D: Costs, Risks, and Rewards. Washington, D.C.: U.S. Government Printing Office; 1993.
10. Noble RC. Education or promotion? [Letter]. N Engl J Med. 1992;327:363.
11. Waud DR. Pharmaceutical promotions—a free lunch? N Engl J Med. 1992;327:351-3.
12. Morelli D, Koenigsberg MR. Sample medication dispensing in a residency practice. J Fam Pract. 1992;34:42-8.

13. Safavi KT, Hayward RA. Choosing between apples and apples: physicians' choices of prescription drugs that have similar side effects and efficacies. J Gen Intern Med. 1992;7:32-7.
14. Accreditation Council for Continuing Medical Education. Standards for commercial support of continuing medical education. Lake Bluff, Illinois: Accreditation Council for Continuing Medical Education; 1992.
15. Code of Pharmaceutical Marketing Practices. Washington, D.C.: Pharmaceutical Manufacturers Association; 1990.
16. Drake DC, Uhlman M. How the drug industry woos doctors. The Philadelphia Inquirer. 14 Dec. 1992, pp. 1 et seq.
17. Berman JL. Physicians and the pharmaceutical industry [Letter]. Ann Intern Med. 1990;113:900.
18. American College of Physicians. American College of Physicians Ethics Manual. Third edition. Ann Intern Med. 1992;117:947-60.

ANNOTATED BIBLIOGRAPHY

Accreditation Council for Continuing Medical Education. Standards for commercial support of continuing medical education. Lake Bluff, Illinois: Accreditation Council for Continuing Medical Education; 1992.

> Offers standards for content, scientific integrity, independence of sponsor, supplementary materials, identification of products, reporting of research results, exhibits, management of commercial funds, disclosure, and financial support of participants in educational activities.

American College of Physicians. Physicians and the pharmaceutical industry. Ann Intern Med. 1990;112:624-6.

> The College's views on gifts and hospitality for physicians, drug industry support of continuing medical education, practitioners and drug trials, and the role of professional societies in this area.

Council on Ethical and Judicial Affairs. Gifts to physicians from industry. JAMA. 1991;265:501.

> The AMA's views on the acceptability of gifts to physicians.

Waud, JR. Pharmaceutical promotions—a free lunch? N Engl J Med. 1992;327:351-3.

> Supports professional persuasion rather than regulation or legislation to encourage appropriate physician behavior and finds that no gift is an acceptable gift, which the author views as a bribe.

Wentz WK, Osteen AM, Gannon MI. Refocusing support and direction. JAMA. 1991;266:953-6; and Continuing medical education: unabated debate. JAMA. 1992;268:1118-20.

> These two articles by CME and credentialing professionals at the AMA chronicle the controversy surrounding industry support of CME and the movement to expand guidelines.

INDEX

125